ABOUT THE AUTHOR

Dr Janet Kennedy is a clinical psychologist practising in New York City. In 2008, Dr Kennedy founded NYC Sleep Doctor, a clinical practice devoted to treating behavioural and psychological sleep problems in babies, toddlers, and adults, and began teaching her popular Raise a Good Sleeper class for new and expectant parents. She spent her early career at the Manhattan VA Medical Center, where she developed a multisite sleep disorders treatment program for veterans. Dr Kennedy lives in Brooklyn with her husband and two children.

The
Good
Sleeper

The
Good
Sleeper

THE ESSENTIAL GUIDE TO SLEEP
FOR YOUR BABY – AND YOU

Dr Janet Kennedy

Vermilion
LONDON

1 3 5 7 9 10 8 6 4 2

Vermilion, an imprint of Ebury Publishing,
20 Vauxhall Bridge Road,
London SW1V 2SA

Vermilion is part of the Penguin Random House group of companies whose
addresses can be found at global.penguinrandomhouse.com

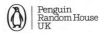

First published by Vermilion in 2015
Published by arrangement with Henry Holt and Company, LLC, 175 5th
Avenue, New York, NY 10011, USA. All rights reserved

www.eburypublishing.co.uk

A CIP catalogue record for this book is available from the British Library

ISBN 9780091954895

Printed in Great Britain by Clays Ltd, St Ives plc

Penguin Random House is committed to a sustainable future for our business,
our readers and our planet. This book is made from Forest Stewardship
Council® certified paper.

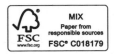

The information in this book has been compiled by way of general
guidance in relation to the specific subjects addressed, but is not a
substitute and not to be relied on for medical, healthcare, pharma-
ceutical or other professional advice on specific circumstances and in
specific locations. So far as the author is aware the information given is
correct and up to date as at January 2015. Practice, laws and regulations
all change, and the reader should obtain up to date professional advice
on any such issues. The author and publishers disclaim, as far as the law
allows, any liability arising directly or indirectly from the use, or
misuse, of the information contained in this book.

For Randy

And for I and L, our two great sleepers

Contents

4. A Schedule Emerges (12–20 Weeks and Beyond)   68

5. Sleeping Through the Night   87

6. Getting Unstuck   117

7. Tricky Circumstances   147

Introduction

Of all the anxieties that plague expecting parents as the due date approaches, fear of sleep deprivation is among the most intense. Everyone knows that the first several weeks are the most difficult. But it is actually what happens after those weeks that determines how well you and your family will function during the first year and beyond.

My clients often ask about my own children. And, yes, they are great sleepers. I was dedicated to shaping their sleep habits from the start, partly because I *needed* them to sleep. I am not one of those people who can function without a decent night's rest.

When I was pregnant with my son, fear of months (or years) of exhaustion inspired me to put together quite a sleep library. At the hospital where I was working, I'd already spent the prior year and a half immersing myself in research to develop a treatment program for adult and geriatric insomnia. While child and adult sleep differ in many ways, certain common principles apply (see Chapter 1). In reading about infant sleep, I was most intrigued by Marc Weissbluth's model of keeping babies well rested and preventing them from becoming overtired. This became the single most important parenting strategy that my husband and I employed.

We tried to ignore the raised eyebrows of friends and relatives who could not believe how much our son was sleeping. I noticed that what often seemed like common sense to me was counterintuitive to others. But soon it became apparent to them that my "trick" was working, and I started helping friends get their kids' sleep on track. Pregnant with my daughter, I began thinking about opening a specialty practice to help other new and expecting parents get off on the right foot. I developed a class called Raise a Good Sleeper and later launched my clinical practice, NYC Sleep Doctor, to work with families stuck in a cycle of bad sleep. Since then, I've helped hundreds of families make simple changes to improve their sleep, and I've supported them through the process of making the difficult ones.

It is my firm belief that good sleepers are not born but

raised. In this book you will find the basic information you need to raise a good sleeper. There are plenty of sleep manuals on the market to guide you through the specifics of various sleep-training strategies. The trouble is, there is no one-size-fits-all technique. Every family is a complex mix of individual temperaments and philosophies. The sheer number of options is overwhelming, deterring many parents from even trying to read up on the subject. And parents who do delve into the literature too often give up because they cannot agree on a strategy or because they don't fully understand the reasoning behind it.

This book is my effort to help people sift through the vast and often confusing information out there and identify strategies that make sense. My goal is to give you a fundamental grasp of infant sleep: how it works, how much is needed, and how to shape good habits. Understanding these principles will help you figure out which strategies will work for you and your family.

In my work, I insist on having parents work together to create a plan. It takes a team effort to stay focused and consistent. I recommend that you read this book together and discuss your priorities and fears *before* the baby is born. Once he or she arrives, you won't have time to read, digest, discuss, plan, or do much more than cope. Of course, your best-laid plans will have to be adjusted and calibrated once your baby arrives. But it is well worth doing the advance planning. The quality of your baby's sleep will have a tremendous impact on your quality of life.

If you did not plan ahead, you certainly aren't alone. Reading sleep manuals is never high on most expecting parents' list of priorities. If you and your child are stuck in a cycle of bad sleep, you are probably doing whatever is necessary just to get through each day and night. But your coping strategies might not be improving the situation—and they could be reinforcing the problem. Once you're mired in it, it's very hard to decide which strategy will lead you out.

Having a good sleeper is not about luck or genes; it is a part of raising a family, and it requires skill, knowledge, and dedication. It is about developing the confidence to identify problems and get back on track quickly.

My children are great sleepers, but they have hit the same bumps in the road that all children do. We have dealt with colic, crying, bedtime battles, early waking, illness, repeated dummy replacement, room-sharing issues, overstimulation, and more. Sometimes we have struggled to know how to respond, but when we make a wrong turn, we go back to the basics and change course. This book will give you those basics, too.

The Good Sleeper Approach
to Infant Sleep

Since opening my private practice, NYC Sleep Doctor, I have entered new parents' homes and lives when they are at their most confused and vulnerable. I have listened to hundreds of exasperated couples as they describe their love for a baby whose sleeplessness is threatening their confidence as parents, their sanity, and even their marriage. They describe how lost they feel as they listen to friendly advice and pore over countless books about sleep. But by the end of our 90-minute visit, they have a firm understanding of what they have missed all along: the simple facts of infant sleep and how to use that knowledge to teach their baby to sleep.

It's not particularly complicated, yet no one seems to have figured out how to explain these concepts and strategies to parents. Pediatricians assess virtually every developmental milestone except sleep. Books, as I will show, are confusing and make promises they can't deliver on. Friends, family, and "parenting coaches" give advice based on their personal experience, which does little to reassure frightened parents who fear doing psychological or physical damage to their child.

In my practice, I have immersed myself in the world of infant sleep—the science and the psychology of it.

When I first started charging fees for my services, I had the usual crisis of confidence: Was I really doing something for these families that they couldn't do themselves? Wasn't this information so straightforward that anyone could figure it out? What I found, as enthusiastic reports came back from parents and as their friends started hiring me, was that what seemed common sense to me was not evident to most parents. I also discovered that I could *transform* the necessary information into common-sense guidelines for my clients.

I spent eight years at the Manhattan Veterans Affairs Medical Center helping patients suffering from arguably the most challenging of sleep issues. Through my experience working with veterans suffering from posttraumatic stress disorder and other serious mental illnesses, I learned how to relate scientific and clinical knowledge to lots of very tough real-life situations. I taught psychology interns how to be concise, responsible writers. I am known among my colleagues and friends as a straight talker—a trait that has gotten me into trouble from time to time but has also been one of my defining professional qualities. My colleagues refer patients to me who need a no-nonsense therapist, one who won't mince words. My presentations are well edited and concise, focusing on the essential points I need to communicate.

I don't use jargon, and I don't try to impress people

with fancy explanations of simple concepts. My goal is to be an effective communicator, and I do that by getting to the point. When I treat my patients, when I teach classes about sleep, or when I lecture students or executives, I typically check in and ask: "Does that make sense?" I do this because I care about my audience, whether it be an individual client, a couple, or a room full of students.

Parents often contact me hoping to put the problem in my hands, expecting me to do something magical to make it disappear. From the beginning, I emphasize that the solution is not magical. My job is to help parents unravel the problem, to determine how and when to intervene, and to arm parents with the knowledge and confidence they need to work through the problem themselves. Parents often ask if I do overnight stays. I don't—and not just because I have my own family. I don't do overnights because parents have to learn how to manage their child's sleep on their own.

I have worked with countless babies with uneventful histories or minor issues like colic. But I have also worked with babies who have had a much harder time: deaf babies, babies who have had neonatal heart surgery or long neonatal intensive care unit stays, and babies and toddlers who have developmental disabilities and serious medical issues. Obviously, special circumstances can affect the methods. But even in these cases, the basic principles apply.

The first things I look for when I'm working with clients are:

1. **The bedtime:** The bedtime is almost always too late. Parents fear that putting their babies to bed too early will cause them to wake up early in the morning. The *exact opposite* is true. An early bedtime is the key to a good night (and reasonable wake-up time).

2. **Naps (where, when, and how long):** Parents often fear that allowing a baby to sleep during the day will compromise night sleep. Most parents do not understand the importance of naps and nap quality.

3. **Short-term survival strategies that are undermining long-term progress:** These can include responding immediately when the baby fusses, co-sleeping, excessive baby wearing, or always waiting to put the baby down fully asleep. Once parents understand their child's process of learning to sleep, they become willing to loosen their grip on survival strategies that are only serving to reinforce the problem.

Another very common problem is the parents' fear of their babies' crying or distress. Parents in some Western countries struggle to foster healthy sleep in their children because they are afraid to allow them to experience distress. They are unable to differentiate between what the child wants and what she needs. Either that, or they simply can't bear to side with the needs over the wants. It's a short-term solution (ending distress or crying by "helping" a baby sleep) that creates a long-term problem (a child that cannot rely on himself to fall asleep independently).

Over the years, I have seen this problem play out in countless ways. There are the men who want to be different from their overbearing fathers and will do anything to avoid "causing" their child distress. There are the parents who coslept with their own parents and recall the difficult transition out of the family bed (when they were old enough to remember); they want to avoid cosleeping but feel judged by their families or peers. There are parents who are essentially traumatized by colic or extreme fussiness in their baby or in an older child and feel unable to tolerate any more crying. There are parents who believe that depriving a child of their attention will create long-term personality defects or even sociopathy (much more on this later). There are parents who fear that they simply don't possess the skills to raise their children effectively, and parents who simply can't agree on a strategy.

Parenting styles naturally shift over the generations in response to changing mores, as well as medical, educational, scientific, and technological advances. But parenting styles also shift as people embrace or reject the merits of their own childhoods. From the late 1960s through the 1980s, the pendulum seems to have swung toward less involved parenting. Society was more focused on self-exploration and fulfillment. As parents made their personal goals and happiness the priorities, the focus on children became less central.

As those children have become the next generation of parents, they have swung the pendulum back, overcorrecting for what they perceive to have been their own parents' disengagement. Many parents today feel compelled to be involved in every aspect of their child's experience, to be omnipresent, to soothe away every discomfort. These are impossible tasks, and they create a lot of problems. **Children who cannot tolerate normal discomforts like boredom, sharing, or having a toy jerked away from them by another baby don't develop the essential life skill that psychologists call distress tolerance.** These children believe they are entitled to be entertained and joyful at all times. Of course, it's important for children to be happy and entertained. But parents' efforts to prevent or soothe away all discomfort teach children that there is something dangerous about being unhappy.

As parents, we all must accept that a child's needs come before his or her wants.

I see it as my job to teach parents that one of the primary challenges they will face is accepting that a child's needs must come before his wants. Clarifying this battle of needs and wants helps parents to understand the challenge at hand. It gives them the courage to begin the task of *parenting*. It gives them permission to prioritize needs and take care of their child's best interest, even when the child is protesting. I teach parents about **authoritative parenting,** which provides the structure to keep the child safe by setting appropriate limits while also allowing the child room to explore and experiment, precisely because he knows that his parents will be there for him if he fails. (Not incidentally, it is this type of parenting that has been found to result in secure attachment and healthy adjustment in the long term.)

The principles and strategies in this book will help you to find a rhythm that brings some sanity to your new life as a parent. The information here will inform your decisions about how to get your baby the sleep she needs while also remaining flexible enough to enjoy your time with your newborn. Countless couples have told me that they wish that someone had explained these things before they became stuck in a cycle of bad sleep. That is precisely what *The Good Sleeper* will do.

CHAPTER 1

It's All About Adrenaline

Everyone knows that babies need a lot of sleep, but most of us still underestimate how much. In the first week or two of life, an infant will sleep up to 18 hours a day. As the weeks roll by, infants gradually spend more time awake, but the average 3-month-old still needs 14–16 hours of sleep per 24-hour period.

It's usually pretty easy to get your baby to sleep during the first couple of weeks. It might even be hard to get a photo of your baby with her eyes open during that time. But after a week or two, your baby will start to wake up more, and she will need your help to make sure that she gets enough sleep.

New parents often assume that babies will naturally fall asleep when they are tired. But the truth is, babies have to learn how to fall asleep. As a parent, you will become your baby's sleep facilitator. By responding to your baby's need to sleep, you will keep your baby well rested and guide her through the process of learning to be a good sleeper.

Adrenaline and Overfatigue

The guiding principle of raising a good sleeper is to **keep your baby from becoming overtired**. The vast majority of sleep problems (and quite a few behavioral problems) have some root in overfatigue.

There is plenty of research on the chemical process that occurs in response to overfatigue, but it boils down to this: When the body becomes overtired, the sympathetic nervous system responds with a release of adrenaline. This is the body's fight-or-flight response, which is a very primitive one. Essentially, if we do not sleep when we are tired, the body presumes that there is a reason for it, some form of problem or threat that requires our attention. The body "helps" out with a burst of energy that keeps us awake. You might notice that when you have been up every 2 hours feeding your infant, it is sometimes difficult to fall asleep at your first opportunity. That's because your own body is hopped up on adrenaline. The same thing happens to babies but in a much more disruptive way.

Babies become overtired quickly, and the adrenaline response is intense. Adrenaline makes it harder for the baby to be soothed or self-soothe, fall asleep, stay asleep, and sleep until a respectable morning hour. Overtired babies fight sleep, wake frequently, and start the day too early. Your job as a parent is to keep your baby from entering this adrenaline-fueled state. Being attentive to your baby's need for sleep and preventing overfatigue can solve sleep problems before they start. A well-rested baby is able to learn how to self-soothe, fall asleep independently, return to sleep during normal night waking, and sleep.

Think about sleep as a 24-hour process. The length and quality of naps and night sleep are connected. Good naps lead to good nights and vice versa. And of course, bad naps and bad nights affect each other, too. You just can't separate day and night sleep. So if your baby is struggling, the task is to figure out when and how to break into the 24-hour loop to get out of the cycle of overfatigue.

Remember: Until your child is well into primary school, whenever you hit bumps with sleep—bedtime battles, night waking, early waking, night terrors, bedtime separation anxiety, nap resistance—step back and figure out when and how your child is becoming overtired. Focusing your attention on the source of overfatigue is the first step to getting back on track.

Of course, it's impossible to avoid overfatigue altogether. It happens to everyone, despite the best intentions.

A baby who occasionally becomes overtired won't struggle too much as long as she is well rested overall. But fatigue accumulates over days and weeks. **A baby who routinely becomes overtired can get stuck in a cycle of poor sleep that wears everyone down.**

Keeping Your Baby Well Rested

Keeping a baby well rested involves two things: watching the clock and watching the baby for drowsiness signs. Paying attention to these will allow you to respond to your baby's need for sleep before she becomes overtired.

Watching the Clock

Babies cannot and should not stay awake for very long. This is critical information, and it contradicts what you will hear from most of your well-meaning family and friends. People tend to believe that babies who sleep too much during the day will not sleep well at night. You must tune folk wisdom out and put your baby to bed frequently. You might not be able to convince the people around you, but if you quietly follow these rules, your critics will see the results.

The truth is, the *more* your baby
sleeps during the day, the better
he or she will sleep at night.

Your baby should not be awake for more than 90 minutes at a time during the first 3 months of life. In fact, your baby might need to sleep again after as little as 1 hour of wakeful time. This might seem crazy, especially if feeding your baby takes a long time (as it can early on). But keeping your baby up longer will result in overfatigue and make it harder for him to get the rest he needs.

The period of wakefulness stretches out after about 3 months, coinciding with longer naps and better nighttime sleep. But even then, watching the clock is critical (more on this later).

Your baby might not *look* tired, especially if she is *over*-tired. Work by the clock anyway. There's no such thing as an 8-week-old baby who needs to stay up for 4 hours. Over time, you will establish a rhythm: your baby will associate a feeling of drowsiness with being soothed to sleep. The more you follow the rule, the easier it becomes to spot when your baby is sleepy and the easier it becomes to help your baby fall asleep.

Following Drowsiness Cues

When your baby is reaching the end of the wakefulness period, he will probably show some signs of drowsiness. If you don't notice any of these signs, start soothing your baby to sleep after about 1 hour and 15 minutes awake.

Babies give subtle cues of drowsiness that are easily

missed. If you learn to recognize them, your baby will get better at letting you know when she is ready to sleep. Over time, you will learn the progression of her cues, and she will learn which of her actions will result in being put down for a nap.

Following drowsiness cues prevents overfatigue because you catch the baby at the optimal time for sleep, before the body releases adrenaline. Adrenaline makes babies seem more awake, making it more difficult to see that they need to sleep. Without the adrenaline to mask the drowsiness, the cues become easier to spot.

One of the first things I ask the parents I work with is what their baby does to tell them she's tired. The most common answer is "She gets fussy." Therein lies the problem: **a fussy baby is already overtired and will fight sleep**.

Instead of waiting for your baby to become uncomfortably tired, look for the subtler cues. If you have trouble identifying them, start tracking how long your baby has been awake when she gets fussy and overtired. Then start watching your baby closely about 15 minutes earlier.

Drowsiness cues are changes in the baby's alertness, activity, and even facial expression. Look for:

- **A pause in activity.** Your baby might be happily engaging with a person or toy—looking, kicking, cooing—and then suddenly she's quiet for a moment. Your baby might re-engage after the pause, but don't be fooled.

- **A single vocalization.** Some babies let out a single squawk or exclamation. This is different from fussiness. It's more like a call to action: imagine your baby saying, "It's time!"

- **The thousand-yard stare.** This often happens during the "pause" described above. Your baby will space out and stare off into the distance. You can almost see her vision blurring. She is clearly less focused.

- **The long, slow-motion blink.** This tends to follow the "thousand-yard stare." Your baby's eyes close slowly and stay shut for longer than the typical blink.

- **Droopy eyes and/or face.** The muscles around the eyes and mouth tend to relax when a baby becomes drowsy.

- **The first yawn.** Don't wait for lots of yawning; the first yawn is a good indication that it's time to go to sleep. (Note, however, that babies often yawn soon after waking up. A good rule of thumb is to attend to yawns that come after your baby has been awake for 1 hour.)

- **"Comfort feeding."** You can tell when your baby is feeding and when he is just sucking for comfort.

Comfort sucking is generally weaker and involves less swallowing. If your baby is comfort feeding and the timing is right, he's probably drowsy. Similarly, less intense dummy sucking can also be an indication of drowsiness.

When you see these signs, start soothing your baby to sleep. Initially, this might involve significant effort, like bouncing, walking, shushing, patting, or even wearing the baby in a carrier. As time goes on, your baby will get used to going to sleep when drowsy, and the routine will become less involved.

If you miss the drowsiness window of opportunity, your baby will become overtired. There are times when it can't be helped and times when it happens so quickly that you're caught by surprise. Don't beat yourself up about it. Just be more vigilant for the next nap, and things will even out.

Here are some signs that your baby is already over-tired:

- **Eye rubbing.** This sign is often mistaken for a drowsiness cue, but it is typically a sign of over-fatigue.
- **Fussiness, crankiness, irritability, whining.**
- **Thrashing around.**

- **Intense effort to nurse but failure to concentrate or settle.**
- **Volatility.** Your baby might be happy one minute, frustrated the next, and then happy again.
- **"Wired" appearance.** Eyes wide open, searching for stimulation/activity, the opposite of sleepy.
- **Bursts of energy.**
- **Putting head down.** This sign is usually followed by jerking the head back up.
- **Clumsiness/sloppiness/loss of coordination.** This triad is more evident in older babies, but it bears mentioning.

If your baby is overtired, all is not lost. You can still soothe your baby to sleep. It's just more difficult, and over time the adrenaline will start to become more disruptive.

Keeping the interval of wakefulness short and responding to drowsiness cues will keep your baby well rested, allowing her sleep to improve naturally as she cruises through the rapid physical and neurological development of infancy. *How* you get your baby to sleep (and even *where* you get her to sleep) depends on her age. During the early weeks, you will be doing most of the work. As time goes on, your baby can learn to do more of her own soothing until she ultimately begins to fall asleep independently. The next chapters will take you through that process step-by-step.

Common Myths and Misconceptions

BABIES WHO SLEEP TOO MUCH DURING THE DAY WILL NOT SLEEP AT NIGHT. *WRONG!* Adult sleep is very different from baby sleep. Adult bodies are programmed to get a certain amount of sleep per 24 hours (7–9 hours). If an adult gets too much sleep during the day, he will get less sleep at night. The priority for adults is to consolidate sleep because nighttime sleep is critical for daytime functioning and health. But naps will help your baby sleep longer at night. The more babies sleep, the better they sleep.

BABIES JUST FALL ASLEEP WHEN THEY'RE TIRED. *WISHFUL THINKING!* In the first couple of weeks, babies sleep easily, and this can lull parents into thinking that the baby will continue to sleep this way. Babies will fall asleep spontaneously *sometimes*, but they will need your help most of the time. Because they transition from drowsy to overtired so quickly, they often miss the opportunity to fall asleep. When parents

> Babies need about twice as much sleep as adults do while their bodies and minds are growing and developing at lightning speed.

respond to drowsiness cues and watch the clock, they intervene when the baby is most easily soothed to sleep, essentially transitioning the baby into sleep instead of allowing the body to take over with the adrenaline response.

Key Points from Chapter 1

- Babies need tons of sleep, but it is hard for them to get the sleep they need when they are overtired.
- Keep in mind that, for at least the first 2–3 months, your baby should not be awake for more than 90 minutes at a time. After that point, he will become overtired.
- The adrenaline release that occurs when your baby is overtired will cause him to fight sleep, sleep fitfully, and wake up before he is fully rested.
- Your baby will show signs of drowsiness before he becomes overtired. Use these as your cue that it is time to start soothing your baby to sleep.

CHAPTER 2

The Early Weeks
(0–6 Weeks Old)

The early weeks of parenthood seem like a blur. So many things are happening at once, and most of them don't happen as planned. The things you expected to be easy end up being harder, and the things that you dreaded fall into place easily. All of those months of reading, researching, nesting, taking classes, and dreaming about life with your baby have passed, and you now have an actual new human being in your home. And you have to figure out how to take care of him or her.

New parents tend to worry about establishing bad sleep habits that will be difficult to break. You will hear a lot about putting the baby down awake, establishing sleep routines, and napping in the cot. However, during the first 6 weeks, your job is to get your baby as much sleep as possible, period. Sometimes that's easier said than done. You will not spoil your baby by soothing him to sleep. Your baby will not become "addicted" to the strategies or tools you're using because you will phase them out *when the time comes.*

You will figure out the strategies that work when your baby is at his best and his worst. When he is at his best, you can work on establishing sleep routines and putting the baby down slightly awake. When he is at his worst, you will do whatever it takes to safely get your baby to sleep. Taking advantage of the easy times will help the fussy, apoplectic times fade away. And as your baby grows and develops the ability to self-soothe more effectively, you can phase out the short-term fixes in favor of good sleep practices.

Where Will Your Baby Sleep?

Safety is your biggest priority when it comes to infant sleep. Sudden Infant Death Syndrome (SIDS) is very real and it's every parent's nightmare. Although there is still much to be learned about SIDS, there are very clear guidelines that dramatically reduce your baby's risk.

Taking these simple steps dramatically reduces your baby's risk for SIDS.

- At night, your baby should sleep in a cot, moses basket, or next to the bed, in a cosleeper—**not in bed with you**. Your bed is a very dangerous place for your baby; it's full of suffocation hazards. Pillows, bed linens, soft mattresses, and sleeping adults are real dangers. You might have heard that breastfeeding mothers are programmed to be aware of their babies next to them and won't roll over on them. *This is simply untrue.* Countless infant deaths have been caused by parents rolling over and inadvertently suffocating their baby.
- Wherever your baby sleeps, the cot mattress should be firm. If you choose to use a cosleeper attached to your bed, make sure to choose one with a firm mattress. Surprisingly, they are not always firm enough.
- Your newborn should sleep on her back.
- Keep toys, blankets, and bumpers out of the cot.
- Do not use a sleep positioner.

New parents often keep the baby in their bedroom for the first several weeks or longer. This is convenient when the baby is still waking frequently for feedings. And new parents often feel more secure having the baby nearby. However, babies make a lot of noise while they sleep. While your baby is sleeping in your room, keep in mind that her noises do not necessarily mean that she is awake.

Take a deep breath and wait a minute or two to see if she is really waking up.

For the first 2–3 months, babies can nap pretty much anywhere. They need a lot of physical contact at this age, so it's normal—and convenient—for babies to nap in your arms or on your body in a carrier of some sort. They also need movement and even noise to re-create the sleep environment they are accustomed to—the womb. As they become more aware of their surroundings—after about 6–8 weeks—sleep quality will be better in the cot, away from the action, but in the early weeks, this matters much less.

During these early weeks, *try* to have the baby nap independently (in a cot, moses basket, swing, etc.) sometimes, both for your own sanity and so he can start to learn to sleep without the constant warmth and smell of you. Right now, you are his primary (perhaps only) sleep cue. Over time, he will get more accustomed to napping without your constant presence, and he will develop other sleep cues. Keep

You will be holding your baby a lot in the first couple of months, and it helps to have a device or two to keep your hands free. Some people swear by slings, and others prefer carriers like the Bjorn or Ergo. Most important when making your choice is to find one that is comfortable for you and keeps your baby safe. If you aren't sure which one to buy, borrow one to have on hand when your baby first comes home and then take your baby with you to a shop to try out various options. Or buy several from a shop with a good return policy so you can test them at home.

in mind that there will be times when it is not possible or desirable for your baby to nap independently. Just try to take advantage of those times when it is more likely to work.

One thing to avoid is napping on the breast. Dozing while feeding is normal at this age, but try not to have the baby nap for longer periods with the breast in his mouth. Clearly, your baby cannot always comfort-feed while sleeping. It is important for her to learn to sleep without constantly feeding, even if it takes some practice. Similarly, **do not prop up a bottle to keep it in your baby's mouth while she is sleeping**. Using a dummy to soothe her will make it easier to put her down for some naps and teach her to sleep more independently.

As babies get older, their sleep quality will start to be compromised when they sleep on you, in motion, in the middle of activity going on around them. This is not the case during the first 6 weeks, so don't worry if your baby won't sleep more than a few minutes after you put her down. Do what works for now, but keep your longer-term goal of more-independent sleep in mind. Each time your baby naps in the cot, she is learning to sleep more independently.

A Hierarchy of Sleep Independence

It helps to keep in mind a sort of **hierarchy of sleep independence**. Over the course of the day, your baby will need more or less help to fall asleep for a particular nap or at bedtime. Work toward using the most independent strategy possible for your baby's needs at that moment.

Following is a list of examples of sleep-soothing strategies in order from most dependent to most independent:

1. Sleeping in arms, on the breast, or while gently holding a dummy in place.
2. Sleeping in arms without sucking or while independently sucking a dummy.
3. Falling asleep in arms and then being transferred to a moving swing.
4. Falling asleep in a swing on high speed or in a stroller in motion.
5. Falling asleep in a vibrating bouncy chair.
6. Falling asleep in a swing on low.
7. Falling asleep in motion or with vibration but having stimulation stopped once asleep.
8. Falling asleep in arms and then being transferred to a motionless, semi-upright device (swing, bouncy seat, infant car seat).
9. Falling asleep in arms then being transferred to a cot or moses basket.
10. Falling asleep in a motionless, semi-upright device.

11. Falling asleep in the cot. This might not happen at all during the first 6 weeks, so don't be alarmed if your baby still needs more help.

Daphne: A Gradual Transition from Arms to Cot

Daphne was 5 weeks old when her mother contacted me for help. Daphne was a very fussy baby and preferred to sleep on her mother. In fact, her mother had not found a way to get Daphne to sleep anywhere else. Needless to say, this was a dangerous situation; Daphne was sleeping in the bed with her exhausted parents, which put her at risk for SIDS. And Daphne's mother was at a breaking point with exhaustion.

Daphne was having a lot of difficulty sleeping comfortably on her back, and because her mother was holding her all the time, she never really got any practice at it. We came up with a gradual solution to help Daphne learn to sleep more independently.

First, Daphne's mum used her own T-shirt to swaddle the baby so she would still be surrounded by her mother's scent even when she was put down. Daphne's mum worked on putting her in her baby swing once she was asleep. Those naps were short at first, so she compensated by holding her for some naps. But Daphne got used to the swing quickly, and her mother was able to put her in it for nights as well. Then she lowered the swinging speed and eventually was able to turn it off once Daphne was in a deep sleep.

By paying close attention to timing and drowsiness cues,

Daphne's mum was preventing the overfatigue that was making it so hard to soothe her. Soon, Daphne was able to fall asleep in the swing instead of being transferred asleep from her mother's arms. Over the next weeks, Daphne's mum worked on putting her into the cot asleep for some naps and then at night. By the time she was 12 weeks old, Daphne was falling asleep in the cot for naps and nights.

Becoming Your Baby's Sleep Facilitator

Your baby will arrive in this world very sleepy. He'll wake up, feed, and go back to sleep. But after a week or two, he'll start spending more time awake. From this point on, begin paying attention to your baby's sleep, watching the clock and watching for drowsiness cues, as described in Chapter 1. The sooner you start doing this, the better. As the weeks go by, you will start to get to know your baby's rhythms, and preventing overfatigue will become more routine. Your baby will get the longest possible stretches of sleep if you keep him from becoming overtired.

At this age, babies need **16 or more hours of sleep per day**. They will get their longest stretch of sleep (up to 4–5 hours) at any time during the day or night. Well-wishers might tell you that you should limit daytime naps so that your baby will sleep her longest at night.

Feeding your baby formula instead of breast milk *will not* improve your baby's sleep. People will tell you that formula takes longer to digest and therefore leads to longer stretches of sleep. In my work, I have not found this to be true. Breast-fed babies' sleep is comparable to that of formula-fed babies.

Thank them kindly, then forget that advice. Your baby might very well get her longest stretch of sleep during the day, but interrupting the long nap won't help her nights. Let her get the sleep she is able to get, whenever that may be. The benefit of being well rested will help her around the clock.

Such long naps are often referred to as "day/night confusion." But your baby's body clock is not actually confused. Simply put, your baby does not have a body clock yet. **Newborns' systems do not start to develop a clock until they are 6–8 weeks old, when melatonin production begins.** Melatonin is one of the hormones that regulates the body's sleep/wake cycle. Cortisol is another hormone involved in this process, helping to establish the body's natural circadian rhythms. Cortisol levels are fairly unpredictable in newborns, and the function of cortisol at this age is somewhat unclear.

You don't need to immerse yourself in infant endocrinology to understand the main point: newborns' sleep is not yet regulated by melatonin. Sleep starts to become much more "organized" after 6–8 weeks, when the body starts to produce the hormone and circadian rhythms begin to emerge. Until that time, your best bet for maximizing nighttime sleep is to keep your baby rested around the clock.

Don't get any ideas about supplementing your baby's melatonin. Remember, melatonin is a hormone. Just because it is deemed "natural" does not mean that it is safe to give to an infant.

As your baby's sleep facilitator, your job is to watch the clock, look for drowsiness cues, and make sure your baby is sleeping frequently. Remember that babies this age should be awake for just 60–90 minutes at a time. Avoiding overfatigue will allow your baby to get her best possible sleep.

Responding to Drowsiness Cues

When you see drowsiness cues, it is time to start soothing your baby to sleep. During the first 6 weeks, that might just mean swaddling your baby and feeding her to sleep. Your baby needs your help falling asleep and, at this stage, almost anything goes. You might do a lot of walking, bouncing, swinging, swaying, or rocking. It really doesn't matter as long as your baby gets to sleep.

But you can also start creating sleep associations or cues that will become signals for sleepiness when repeated over time. To create sleep associations, simply pair other cues with the things that work. Sing a

Sleep associations develop through a process called **classical conditioning.** Pavlov's dog learned that every time a bell was rung, he would be fed. Eventually, he would start salivating when he heard the bell *even when there was no food.* Similarly, your baby will learn to relax in response to cues that you create. Rocking your baby helps her to relax. Singing while rocking will teach your baby to relax when sung to.

particular song while you are breast-feeding or rocking your baby to sleep. The song will become a sleep cue over time and your baby will begin to relax when he hears it. Routines and sleep cues will become more important in the next phase of development, but you can—and should—start introducing them right away.

As you and your baby get into a rhythm of his falling asleep when he becomes drowsy (instead of overtired), it can become easier to soothe your baby. This might not happen yet, but when it does, you can start to teach your baby to be less reliant on being fed to sleep. Simply stop feeding when the baby has finished, before he does much comfort sucking (you'll know because there will be less swallowing). Then soothe your baby to sleep another way—rocking, walking, singing, swaying—anything that works. If your baby seems pleasantly calm and drowsy, you can also try putting him in the cot awake and patting or shushing him until he falls asleep. Or let him fuss for a few minutes to see if he can fall asleep independently. Most babies don't do much of this during the first 6 weeks; but if you see an opportunity, give it a try. If your baby is unable to fall asleep, you can pick him up again and soothe him to sleep.

White Noise

White noise is an important sleep cue and soothing tool. Newborns are used to sleeping in the womb, which is a pretty noisy environment. Quiet rooms don't do much to help them sleep. (In fact, your newborn might sleep better in a crowded restaurant.) White noise can re-create that sensation and blanket the room with a comforting shushing. I recommend plain white noise rather than oceans, heartbeats, rain forest sounds, or the like. Plain white noise is the most neutral. I also prefer to use nondigital white noise—a machine that essentially has a small fan in a case—rather than a digital sound machine because the sound is more pleasant and seems to buffer extraneous noise better. Don't blast white noise in your baby's ears or place the machine immediately next to the cot. The best spots tend to be near the window (to buffer outside noise) or near the door (to buffer noise in your home). White noise should stay on all night and through naps (at least the ones that happen in the bedroom).

> I don't often recommend specific products. But when it comes to white noise, I truly prefer the machine made by Marpac Dohm, often called the Sleep Mate or "dual speed sound conditioner."

Responding to Night Waking

One of the hardest parts of the first 6 weeks is the amount of tending that babies need during the night. Babies wake up because they are hungry or because they have completed a sleep cycle and have woken fully instead of transitioning back to deep sleep. Your baby still needs to eat several times per night, and she doesn't yet have the ability to self-soothe. When your baby wakes up during the night, take care of business and get her back to sleep. Keep the lights off or very low. Do not engage with your baby by talking, playing, or making much eye contact. And keep the stimulation to a minimum. Over time, your baby will start to recognize these nighttime cues, and the length of her nighttime wakefulness will shorten.

As the weeks pass, start allowing your baby a little more time to fuss before you go to him in the night. Often, babies do not learn to self-soothe because parents respond to them too quickly. Giving your baby a minute—or several—to settle himself will teach him how to return to sleep. It won't work every time. Sometimes your baby will wake up fully and need to be fed; other times, he might grunt and snort a bit without fully waking and then settle back into deeper sleep.

Parents often fear that if they let the baby wake fully during the night it will be harder to get her back to sleep.

That might be the case *occasionally,* but giving your baby the chance to return to sleep before you spring into action (or, more likely, drag yourself into action) will help her to gradually lengthen her stretches of sleep. Every time your baby settles herself, she is *learning how to self-soothe.* Allowing this process to evolve gradually can lead to sleeping through the night without long bouts of crying. It doesn't always work so smoothly, but it is often very effective.

Dummies

Babies need to suck, and at this age, they aren't coordinated enough to really take advantage of their hands. Dummies are controversial in some circles, but I am a firm believer in them. Unless you are having lactation problems, using a dummy won't disrupt breastfeeding or cause nipple confusion. Anyone who has breastfed a newborn for an hour, only to have him start smacking his lips 10 minutes later knows that not all sucking is about feeding. **Dummies have also been found to decrease the risk of SIDS.**

Dummies fulfill the sucking need, and it is worth making a real effort to get your baby to take one. Forget about your fear of having a four-year-old with a dummy. Most babies stop using the dummy naturally. Those who don't can give it up—with a little suffering—when the need to suck starts to diminish. But right now, your baby needs to suck. And you need a break. *Give that baby a dummy.*

Babies don't necessarily love dummies from the start. If your baby won't take one, try pulling it out gently. That often prompts a baby to suck it in instead of spitting it out. Keep trying.

The Onset of Fussiness

Sometime around 2 weeks of age, babies tend to develop a daily period of fussiness, typically in the evening. This fussy period usually lasts 2–3 hours and is at its worst when your baby is about 6 weeks old. After that, it tends to diminish and disappear altogether by 10–12 weeks. The precise cause of the fussiness is not known, but it is now clear that it is not related to gastrointestinal distress, as was once thought. It is essentially just another developmental phase, albeit not a very pleasant one for you or your baby.

Coping with Colic

During this period of fussiness, the baby appears unsettled and uncomfortable. More heroic efforts are required to soothe him, and he's certainly not offering up social smiles. There is a continuum of fussiness, with so-called easy babies at one end and full-blown colic at the other. Colic is defined as a period of crying that lasts more than 3 hours, occurring more than 3 days per week for more than 3 weeks *in an otherwise healthy and well-fed baby.*

Fussiness does not have to ruin your baby's sleep development. **Look at the fussy hours as a discrete period separate from the rest of the day.** Follow all of the sleep facilitator rules for the 21 or 22 nonfussy hours and then do whatever is necessary to get through the challenging hours.

David: Keeping a Colicky Baby Rested

David was 6 weeks old when his mother attended my Raise a Good Sleeper class. David's two older siblings had been "bad sleepers," and his mum was determined to do things differently. The trouble was that David had colic. His daytime naps were erratic, and overfatigue was making matters worse. Each night at 7 p.m. David would become inconsolable. His mother could not put him down without hysterics, but she was afraid that holding him was fostering bad habits. Things were particularly difficult because David's witching hour coincided with her older kids' evening routines.

Based on David's mother's description, it was clear that the 7 p.m. meltdown was different in quality from the fussiness or overfatigue that occurred at other times during the day. I encouraged her to consider the colicky time as distinct from the rest of the day, doing what was necessary to keep David calm and

A person could go broke buying all of the various items designed to soothe colicky babies. In my day, which wasn't that long ago, options were limited to your basic bouncy seat with or without vibration, swings, and what was then revolutionary, a vibrating rocker. Nowadays, there are seats that rotate in a million directions and every variety of expensive necessity. When your baby is colicky, you are desperate, and so you will buy anything that promises relief. These things might help somewhat, but your baby is still going to need lots of hands-on soothing from you. And he will still cry. There is no perfect device. Arm yourself with a couple of options and remember that this will all pass in a few weeks.

working on establishing good sleep habits for the rest of the day. The relief David's mum felt was palpable. Each night, his colicky hours had undermined her confidence in her ability to foster healthy sleep in her child, and she began to dread the return of long years of sleep deprivation ahead of her. But now she was able to step back and form a plan of action, one that included getting temporary help in the evenings until David's colic subsided.

Parents often worry that what they do to soothe a colicky baby will create bad habits. The best way to avoid that is to create good habits when your baby is in a good state. If your baby is well rested for the vast majority of the day, she'll rebound more easily when she grows out of the colicky phase.

There are two common ways in which this strategy goes wrong: parents continue heroic soothing efforts around the clock, even when the baby doesn't

need them, and parents don't recognize when the baby has grown out of colic and is simply overtired.

Tips for Coping with Colic

1. Look for a pattern and plan around it. If your baby is a mess at 6 p.m. every day, don't plan to cook dinner, talk to your mother on the phone, or do much of anything at that time. Freeze dinners, order in, or bring in a local teenager to help. Accept that this is happening. If you are blindsided by fussiness every evening, you will be even more miserable.

2. Line up an arsenal of tools to help soothe your baby. Chances are, motion or vibration will have to be involved. There are swings, bouncy chairs or rockers that vibrate, exercise balls to bounce on. Make sure that you have several choices in rotation.

3. Work as a team with your partner. Remember that this is a phase. It is not an indication of your baby's temperament or the amount of crying you have in store for the next eighteen years. Plan for each of you to take the baby in shifts. **Also keep in mind that it's often easier for the non-breastfeeding partner to soothe the baby in this state because the smell of milk on the breastfeeding mother triggers a desire to feed even when the baby does not need feeding.**

4. Watch Harvey Karp's *Happiest Baby on the Block* video (see "Suggested Reading and Viewing") to learn the five *S*'s and see some magical strategies in action. I used these strategies with my own kids, and they made a huge difference. Dr. Karp believes that, compared to other mammals, human infants are born underdeveloped and spend the first 3 months of life essentially completing their prenatal development. He refers to the first 3 months of life as the "fourth trimester," and his five *S*'s are essentially tools to re-create the sensations experienced in utero.

5. Swaddle your baby even if he fights it. This is part of the five *S*'s, but it is worth its own bullet point. Newborns sleep much better when they are swaddled. Chances are, you will never be able to swaddle your baby as well as the neonatal nurses did in the hospital. Fortunately, there are plenty of foolproof swaddle blankets with special wrapping techniques or Velcro fasteners to assist the swaddle challenged.

6. Use a dummy. The dummy is an important tool for helping your baby settle down. If your baby rejects the dummy, keep trying.

7. Don't plan to put your baby down much during the fussy hours unless you need to take a break as

described below; your colicky baby will need virtually constant attention to remain calm. When the fussy time passes, your baby will be able to sleep.

8. Take a break. If you are getting frustrated, put your baby down in a safe place and walk away for a few minutes. Your baby can cry unattended for a few minutes while you take some deep breaths and compose yourself.

9. Say yes to all offers of help. Anything that takes something off your list or allows you some breathing room will make a difference.

10. Take care of yourself during the easier hours. Nap when you can. Eat well. Shower and put on real clothes. Call friends. Get out of the house at least once a day.

11. Never, ever shake your baby.

Is It Reflux?

Reflux gets a lot of attention these days. Newborns often have some form of reflux as their gastrointestinal systems mature. However, most babies do not need reflux medication, special formula, or the elimination of dairy or gluten from the breastfeeding mother's diet. Colic is often misinterpreted by parents as reflux, and doctors respond to parents' distress with prescriptions for acid reducers.

Studies show that these medications are overprescribed for infants. However, there are certainly plenty of babies who need medication, elimination diets, and/or special formula. Symptoms of acid reflux in infants include:

- Poor weight gain
- Spitting up forcefully, causing stomach contents to shoot out of the baby's mouth (projectile vomiting)
- Spitting up green or yellow fluid
- Spitting up blood or a material that looks like coffee grounds
- Refusing food
- Blood in the stool
- Difficulty breathing

Avoid Information Overload

Parents often engage in endless searching for *the strategy* that will make all of this easy. The fact is, the first couple of months of parenthood are hard—wonderful but really hard. Resist the impulse to read everything available. Resist the urge to spend hours doing Internet searches or chatting on message boards. You should be well informed, but at a certain point, you will just be spinning your wheels, wasting your time, and undermining your confidence.

Key Points from Chapter 2

- The first 6 weeks are challenging. You will be in survival mode a lot of the time.
- You cannot create bad habits, but you can work on good habits some of the time.
- Keeping your baby well rested will make it easier for him to fall asleep, stay asleep, and get the rest that he needs.
- Your baby does not yet have a body clock, so sleep will be unpredictable.
- Waking your baby from long naps will not produce longer sleep at night. More daytime sleep is the best way to achieve more nighttime sleep.
- Follow drowsiness cues and make sure your baby is not awake for more than 90 minutes at a time.
- Arm yourself with tools and strategies to soothe your baby's fussiness.
- Start waiting a few minutes when your baby makes noises at night to see if he is truly awake and in need of something.

CHAPTER 3

The Light at the End of the Newborn Tunnel (6–12 Weeks)

Several years before I had my first child, I was visiting with a close friend and her newborn daughter when her mother-in-law offered these words of wisdom about the early weeks of motherhood: "For the first four weeks it's like you're a slave to a stranger." That advice stuck with me, maybe because of her unforgettable Rhode Island accent, but more likely because it was the first time I had heard anyone speak honestly about the drudgery that goes along with the wonder of caring for a newborn. The fact is, in the first month, babies don't give a whole lot back.

But as they reach the 6-week mark, a lot starts to change. Among other things, you have a much better sense of how to soothe your baby, your body is starting to feel human again after childbirth, and your baby knows you're alive. Sometime between 4 and 12 weeks of age, your baby will start smiling at you, and it feels like the clouds are parting.

With this social awareness comes a new desire to engage. Babies who could sleep anywhere suddenly struggle to fall asleep in the middle of the action. They start to fight sleep to be with you. And they start to become more stimulated by your presence. When this happens, it becomes even more important to pay attention to your baby's drowsiness cues. Your baby might be having a better time being awake, but she still needs a lot of sleep. In fact, protecting and facilitating your baby's naps and night sleep will allow her to sleep longer and better, easing her into natural sleep rhythms and allowing her to develop the ability to self-soothe.

The Beginnings of the Body Clock

Sometime between 6 and 8 weeks of age, the natural bio-rhythm regulating sleep and wakefulness starts to evolve as the body begins to produce melatonin. At this point, your baby's longest stretches of sleep will start to come reliably at night. If you continue to pay attention to drowsiness cues and make sure your baby is not awake for more than 90 minutes at a time, your baby's nighttime sleep will benefit even more. **Remember: There's no such thing as "too much" daytime sleep.**

Now that your baby's melatonin is beginning to work for him, it becomes more important for the baby to sleep in a dark room. Light—even artificial light—will interfere with the release of melatonin. **Make sure the bedroom is very dark and use a dim night-light when you go to the baby in the night.** Keeping stimulation to a minimum during the night also reinforces the difference between day and night, teaching your baby to sleep for longer uninterrupted stretches.

Exposure to light at the right times also helps to set your baby's body clock. When your baby gets up for the day, open the blinds and expose him to daylight. This suppresses melatonin and starts the daytime body clock in motion. When it is time for naps, make it dark again. This contrast helps the natural biorhythm—and with it, predictable, restorative sleep—to develop.

As your baby's biorhythm develops, bedtime will naturally begin earlier. At some point between 8 and 12 weeks of age, your baby will need to start going to bed before 8 p.m. Babies and young children produce levels of melatonin much higher than those of adults, creating a natural bedtime in the early evening. As melatonin levels climb at the end of the day, babies become drowsy. This is the body's signal that it is time to slow down and sleep for an extended, restorative period. Keeping your baby up too late will start to interfere with his ability to sleep for longer stretches at night because he will have to fight to stay awake through his body's natural bedtime. Parents often try to keep the baby up to get the longest stretch of night sleep when they want to sleep themselves. But this will backfire—probably sooner than later—and the baby will become too tired to sleep well.

Six weeks also marks the peak of infant fussiness or colic. Fussiness gradually diminishes over the next 4–6 weeks. Keeping your baby rested during the nonfussy hours will help this process and allow your baby to rebound quickly when he ages out of this normal fussiness.

The Sleep and Eating "Schedule"

Keeping your baby rested is still the priority. Your baby will sleep better, eat better, and be happier in general if she is well rested. By this point, you and your baby are probably developing your own language, and it is easier for you to recognize drowsiness cues. If your baby is not the greatest communicator, watch the clock instead. Your baby still can't stay up more than about 90 minutes without becoming overtired; and an overtired baby is less able to learn how to sleep independently. If your baby's naps remain short, she might nap five or six times a day. As her biorhythm starts working for her, the naps will lengthen and consolidate.

Parents often worry about how to keep a baby on a feeding schedule and still prioritize sleep. Sleep and feedings don't always coordinate perfectly, and parents have to decide what to do. I make sleep the priority *unless* there is a feeding issue that takes precedence. If there is any reason that you must keep to a strict feeding schedule (weight, feeding issues, lactation concerns, or other medical issues), just do your best with sleep and work on it more aggressively when the more pressing issue resolves. If your doctor wants you to wake the baby to feed, do it.

But if there is no other pressing issue, bump sleep to the top of the list. Your baby will still feed on a schedule; it will just be a more flexible one. There will be times when your baby is drowsy 90 minutes after a feeding and then takes a 2-hour nap. If your baby is on a 3-hour feeding schedule, she will be sleeping through her usual feeding time. But don't wake her at the scheduled feeding time. She'll feed when she wakes up. Sometimes, you'll be feeding a bit before or a bit after the scheduled feeding time.

Unless it's close to the time for a feeding, try not to feed right before the nap. **Avoiding the feed/sleep association will help your baby learn to fall asleep**

on her own. It will be easier to put her down if she is not used to falling asleep on the breast or bottle each time. Feeding right before naps also increases the likelihood that wind, spit-up, or reflux will interfere with the nap.

As naps lengthen, you will settle into more of what's known as the "sleep-eat-play" schedule. Your baby will wake up in the morning and feed. She'll go down for the first nap before the next feeding time and she'll wake up hungry. You'll feed soon after she wakes up from each nap. The only feeding before sleep will be during the routine at bedtime.

David, Part 2: Balancing Feeding and Sleep Schedules

David, whose mother attended my class when he was 6 weeks old, was much less colicky when his mother contacted me a few weeks later. But she was concerned about balancing his feeding and sleeping schedule. Taking a look at David's sleep schedule, it was clear that his naps were too far apart. He was getting over-tired before the first nap, and as a result, that nap was not lengthening. He ended up cluster feeding or snacking throughout the day, which was becoming difficult to manage with two other kids in the house.

I suggested that David's mum put him down for the first nap sooner, after just 60–90 minutes awake. David would feed after waking for the day and then not again until after his first nap. As his first nap lengthened to 90 minutes and then to 2 hours, he woke rested—and hungry for a full meal. Once his feedings consolidated, his night waking diminished, too, likely because he had consumed enough of his calories during the day. Eventually, David began sleeping through the night on his own, simply because his naps and daytime feeding consolidated.

The Sleep Environment

Your baby is starting to pick up on cues from the environment. He is more easily stimulated (and overstimulated), and his stretches of uninterrupted sleep during the day and at night could be lengthening. It is time to pay more attention to where, when, and how your baby is sleeping.

Your baby might still be in the throes of colic for several hours a night or she might nap much better in your arms at certain times of day. Do not worry about the things you are still doing to get by at your baby's most challenging moments. But when your baby is at her best, you can start to ease into more consistent independent sleep.

Start to protect your baby's sleep by having him nap at home at least some of the time. By the time he reaches 12 weeks, the quality of his sleep will be compromised by light, noise, and motion. He will be much better rested if he sleeps motionless, in the dark, and without the stimulating smell and feel of you or someone else holding him. Weeks 6–12 give you the opportunity to work toward more independent sleep without giving up the fail-safe strategies that still work for the short term.

Easing into Independent Napping

Start establishing sleep cues by bringing your baby into the bedroom for the soothing process, making it dark, swaddling her, and turning on white noise. Initially, you will be soothing your baby to sleep and then putting her down. But when you sense that she is in a good state— drowsy but still awake—try putting her in the cot.

Strategies for easing into cot napping at the end of the routine:

- If your baby sleeps mostly in motion, move the swing into the bedroom. That way, she will have the established cue (swing/motion) that works while developing new cues (bedroom, dark, white noise). Over time, slow down the swing and then turn it off altogether. Once she is used to napping motionless in her room, you can work on the cot.
- As an alternative to the swing, you can use a rocking moses basket in the bedroom. When you put

your baby down, you will be able to rock the moses basket gently to help her fall asleep. As she gets used to falling asleep in the moses basket instead of in your arms, you can phase out the rocking.

• Put her in the cot drowsy but awake and pat her, stroke her face, sing to her, or rub her head until she is asleep. Whatever soothing strategy works will become a sleep cue. Over time, you will be able to use the strategy to help her stay calm when you put her in the cot. But you will be able to stop *before* she is asleep and leave her to fall asleep independently.

• Put her in the cot drowsy but awake, do something soothing as described above, and leave. If she fusses, give her some time to work it out. If she really cries, go in, pick her up, and get her calm. Then put her back in the cot. If this fails several times, pick her up and soothe her to sleep, but try again for the next nap.

• Put her down in the cot drowsy but awake, do something soothing, and leave. Let her cry for 5 minutes. Go in, pick her up, soothe her until calm and put her down again. Let her cry for another 5–10 minutes. Repeat. If she doesn't sleep, get her up and wait until the next nap. This level of crying will not harm your infant. This is not full "cry-it-out" or what is also known as extinction. This is experimenting with giving your baby the opportunity to fall asleep independently.

> Parents are often afraid or reluctant to let their babies cry at all. As a result, they have no idea whether 5 minutes of crying would teach their baby how to nap.

I often hear from parents of 3- and 4-month-old babies that the baby does not sleep well in their arms, but she also doesn't know how to sleep in the cot. There will come a time when your baby is so stimulated by you that she can't easily fall asleep in your arms (and possibly even in your presence). Teaching her to sleep alone prior to that point will ease the transition. In other words, the time has come to put the baby down.

When babies learn to fall asleep independently, they also develop the ability to return to sleep independently. Naps lengthen past 45 minutes because the baby is able to return to sleep independently after one sleep cycle. Likewise, nighttime stretches of sleep lengthen as well.

Establishing the Bedtime Routine

The bedtime routine is one of the most important parts of the day. It tells your baby that it is time to settle down and go to sleep. Using consistent bedtime cues will train your baby's body to relax and become drowsy as the routine progresses. The elements of the bedtime

Parents often fear that their baby has inherited a sleep problem from them. But the vast majority of infant sleep problems are behavioral, not genetic or even physiological. By teaching your baby to sleep, you are giving him a lifelong skill.

routine will evolve over the months and years. But the ritual of quieting down with you before bed will teach your child how to create a real separation between daytime and night. That's something adults often don't do very well for themselves.

Some parents want to avoid a routine because they don't want to be tied to it. But the routine doesn't have to be an elaborate, time-consuming ordeal. It's simply a predictable progression that ends in sleep.

The bedtime routine starts when you enter the bedroom with your baby. You can give your baby a bath if he needs one, but the bath is not essential to the routine.

- When you go into your baby's room, close the door behind you.
- Dim the lights.
- Turn on soft music if you use it.
- Definitely turn on white noise.
- Get the baby changed into pajamas.
- Give a massage if you want.
- Sit down and feed the baby.
- Stop feeding when the baby is just sucking for comfort (weaker sucking, less swallowing).

- Hold the baby and do something else like sing, hum, or rock so that the baby doesn't associate feeding with sleep.

The next step depends on where you are in the process of teaching your baby to fall asleep. You might still be putting your baby down asleep. As the weeks go by, start putting her in the cot more awake and soothing her there until she falls asleep. Then work on soothing her in the cot to help her make the transition but stopping while she is still awake and letting her fall asleep on her own. You can also experiment with letting her fuss or cry for 5–10 minutes at a time.

> The cot is no place for a bottle—ever. Putting your baby into the cot with a bottle is a bad idea at every age. There are real health risks such as tooth decay—even before your baby has teeth—and ear infections. And it reinforces the sleep/feeding association that interferes with your baby's ability to self-soothe.

Lengthening Night Sleep

Babies make a lot of noise during the night, and a parent's instinct is to respond as quickly as possible. Parents often *purposely* intervene before the baby wakes fully because it seems easier to get the baby back to sleep. The trouble is, your baby doesn't need you to respond to every snort, fuss, or shout. And if you do spring into action each time you hear something, you will wake your baby unnecessarily, and you will keep her from learning how to transition through a shift in sleep cycle *without* your help.

In the beginning, it is hard to hold back. You are exhausted and you rationalize that feeding the baby *now* will let you get more sleep. You're already awake, and you don't know how long it will be before your baby wakes up for a feeding. If you feed her right away, you know you'll buy yourself at least a couple of hours of sleep. Sometimes it's just too hard to wait it out. That's fine! Just keep this in mind and, as you can, start giving the baby more time to settle before intervening.

The period between 6 and 12 weeks is also a good time to move the baby out of your bedroom.* As night

---

* In 2011 the American Academy of Pediatrics published updated safety recommendations for SIDS prevention. They recommend that infants sleep in the room with parents but not in the same bed *for the first year*. They note that room sharing allows easier access to the baby for nighttime soothing and feeding without the risks associated with bed sharing. However, based on my reading of the available literature, the benefit of this longer-term room sharing in SIDS prevention is not well demonstrated. In the UK, the NHS SIDS advice suggests that your baby should sleep in the same room but not the same bed as you until 6 months old.

The original literature cited in these recommendations does not adequately isolate the effect of room sharing on SIDS risk reduction. In one study, the vast majority of infant deaths involved sleeping on the side or belly, positions known to increase the risk of SIDS. In another study, the elevated risk of sleeping in a separate room was present only for babies whose mothers were smokers. Thus the recommendation for longer-term room sharing may be overly conservative.

However, when you do move your baby into a separate room for sleep starts to lengthen, you won't be feeding your baby as frequently. Getting out of bed starts to feel possible when you are getting longer stretches of sleep yourself and when your baby is down to feeding just a couple of times during the night. Moving the baby out of your room has several advantages:

- *You will sleep better.* Babies make a lot of noise while they are sleeping. New mothers are wired to respond viscerally when their babies are unsettled. With the baby farther away from you, you will be able to sleep through some of the baby's sleep noises and wake up only when he actually needs you.
- *You won't wake your baby unintentionally.* A certain "mum vibe" exists between you and your baby. Your hyperalertness to your baby's sleep noise can actually wake your baby up. You might physically wake your baby by responding as though he is awake. Your baby is also sensitive to your presence. Nearby, he can smell you, hear you, and possibly see you. Farther away from you, he is less likely to wake fully.

---

sleeping, it is absolutely necessary to address all other SIDS risk factors. Make sure the cot is safe and always put your baby down to sleep on her back. If your baby has any known physiological risk factors for SIDS, discuss with a doctor whether it is safe to discontinue room sharing.

- *Your baby will get to practice self-soothing.* In the time it takes you to realize that the baby is awake, drag yourself out of bed, and get to the baby, he might just get himself back to sleep.

Moving your baby out of your room is an emotional milestone. I recall standing over my son's cot the first night, manufacturing reasons to bring him back into my room. After all, this baby had been part of my body for a long time: through pregnancy, many hours in the baby carrier or my arms, and feeding. Realizing this separation is naturally bittersweet, but we're talking about sleep here. And the bottom line is that your baby will sleep better with some distance.

If you just aren't ready to move your baby out of the bedroom, consider moving him farther away from you. Put the side up on your cosleeper and move it across the room. Move the moses basket to the other side of the bed. And restrain yourself when your baby makes noise during the night. **Make sure he is really awake before you go to him.**

Baby Monitors

Baby monitors, especially video monitors, are a mixed blessing. On the one hand, it's reassuring to be able to hear or see your baby without getting up or possibly disturbing her. Video monitors in particular allow parents to check on the baby surreptitiously. That can be very helpful when you are trying to determine whether your baby is awake. But it can easily turn into something less helpful: a *need* to check on the baby excessively.

The fact is you don't need to hear or see every peep or movement your baby makes when she is alone in her cot. The cot, after all, is a safe environment free of all choking and suffocation hazards (and, later, climbing hazards). Constant monitoring can lead to a type of hypervigilance that interferes with your baby's sleep. When you hear your baby, your body tells you that you should *do* something. But rushing to do something prevents your baby from learning to self-soothe.

Your hypervigilance interferes with your baby's sleep.

Unless you are unable to hear your baby's full-throated cry from your bedroom, you do not need to keep a baby monitor on all night. Turning it off will allow you to sleep through the minor waking that occurs through the night. Either your baby will self-soothe and go back to sleep, or he will wake fully and make his presence known. You will hear your baby when he needs you. By all means, if using a monitor is the only way you can tolerate moving your baby to another room, use it. But ease yourself out of it as you get used to being away from your baby.

Transitioning to the Cot

Newborns like to be in snug sleep environments, but they will have to transition to a cot sooner or later. As they get bigger and start squirming around more, a moses basket or cosleeper is going to be too cramped. Parents fret over this transition, but it isn't typically that much trouble.

- Start with naps so your baby gets used to being in the cot.
- Don't use a freshly laundered swaddle. It helps the baby to have the familiar smell of last night's swaddle blanket.
- If your baby is already able to fall asleep in the moses basket after being put down slightly awake, you can put the moses basket in the cot for a few nights and then put the baby straight in the cot.
- If you are moving your baby out of your room at the same time, use the cosleeper in his room for a few nights before trying the cot.
- Keep other sleep cues consistent (e.g., white noise, darkness, "your" song).

Making the transition to the cot sooner rather than later is a good idea. As babies approach the 3-month mark, they are developing stronger sleep associations. If the bigger changes happen when they are still less aware of their surroundings, it can be much easier.

Dummies

Yes, dummies fall out. Before your baby is old enough to sleep through the night, you can replace the dummy when your baby starts fussing. **Do not use anything to artificially secure a dummy in your baby's mouth.** As your baby gets older, she will learn that spitting out the dummy gets your attention. At that point, she will have to learn to sleep without it if she spits it out.

Not all night waking is about hunger. If your baby has been fed fairly recently, try using the dummy to get her back to sleep instead of feeding. If it fails, you can always feed. But spacing out the feedings this way can lead to fewer night wakings.

Swaddles

Swaddles are still important at this age even though babies start to fight them more. At 6 weeks, babies are still making a lot of jerky movements in their sleep and

As with everything baby-related these days, there is a huge market for specialized swaddle blankets. This is one area where your money will be well spent. Gone are the days when you had to learn the art of baby burrito making. No matter how easy it looked, I could never get that last tuck to stay. The day I discovered a special swaddle blanket was indeed a happy one! Some babies need extreme swaddling, whereas others simply need a blanket with a little Velcro. One mum I know had a little Houdini and resorted to duct-taping the swaddle blanket. It's worth trying a couple of varieties to find one that's best for your baby.

end up slapping themselves awake. Most babies still need the tight, confined feeling of the womb to sleep well. If your baby calms easily and sleeps well without the swaddle, there's no need to force it. But if your baby is fighting the swaddle, try a tighter one before giving up, especially if your baby is very fussy or colicky.

As the weeks roll on, your baby will become more interested in his hands. This is the beginning of self-soothing. Babies often begin sucking on their hands instead of looking for a breast or bottle. As this starts to happen, the swaddle can be phased out. You can try leaving one arm out at first. Or try one nap at a time without the swaddle as you build up to unswaddling at night. If your baby is very dependent on swaddling and you plan to use crying to teach her to sleep through the night, don't bother phasing out the swaddle. Just wait until your baby is ready for cry-it-out and do it all at once.

By the time your baby is 12–16 weeks, she should not be using the swaddle. Once your baby can roll over, the swaddle becomes dangerous. Your baby needs to be able to push up with her hands to reposition herself. Similarly, I feel strongly that you should not use a swaddle when doing full cry-it-out.

Sleep sacks are optional. They don't really approximate the feeling of being in a swaddle, so they aren't of much use as you teach your baby to sleep unbound. Some babies don't mind sleep sacks, and they become a sleep cue as part of the bedtime routine. Other babies get frustrated with the sleep sack as they learn to move around at night and reposition themselves. Certainly, if your baby is sleeping in a very cold room and needs a blanket, a sleep sack is the way to go. Otherwise, it's harmless but unnecessary.

Challenging Situations: Colic and Reflux

If your baby has colic or reflux, you are probably feeling pretty discouraged by this chapter. Your baby seems nowhere near ready for these strategies. It's true, these are very challenging situations and your baby will have a harder time self-soothing. You might not be able to put your baby down much at all for sleep. You are in survival mode. (And I know: I went through it with my daughter.) Don't feel guilty about it. And don't compare yourself to others who are having an easier time of it. But do get yourself some support. Colic is essentially the extreme version of normal fussiness. It occurs during a discrete time of day. It tends to come on like a freight train and turn off like a light. Try to keep track of it from day to day so you can figure out your baby's rhythms. For example, if your baby explodes with colic between 9 p.m. and midnight, she will need near-constant attention during that time. That means bouncing, rocking, helping with the dummy, swinging, shushing, etc. She might be relatively calm while you do these things, but she'll get quite upset if you stop and try to put her down. Once you realize that this is the pattern, stop trying to get her to sleep during that time of night. She will fall asleep once her colicky time passes. If you spend those hours trying to get her to sleep and putting her down, you will become depressed and demoralized. Instead, do what you have to do to get through the trying hours. During the rest of the day, the strategies described in this chapter can work for your baby.

Reflux is a different story. It doesn't tend to be isolated to specific times of day. Talk to your doctor about appropriate treatment. That might include medication, or it might just include changes to what, when, and how you feed the baby. It can be much harder to soothe a baby who has reflux, but it's important to avoid constantly feeding for comfort because it can create more stomach discomfort. When it comes to sleep, do your best with the strategies above. Keep them in mind, but don't worry if you just can't make it work. Your priority is getting through this tough time, and if your baby doesn't learn to fall asleep independently right now, you can teach him later.

Key Points from Chapter 3

- Your baby's body clock starts to develop between 6 and 12 weeks as melatonin production begins.
- Keeping your baby well rested allows his or her body clock to develop naturally.
- Continue following drowsiness cues and keeping the interval of awake time short (90 minutes).
- Establishing bedtime routines helps your baby to learn how to self-soothe.
- Transitioning to sleeping at home, in the cot, and farther away from you will improve sleep quality and foster more self-soothing.
- Putting your baby into the cot before she is fully asleep will lessen her reliance on you (and feeding) for sleep. It will also help to lengthen sleep, as your baby will be more able to return to sleep independently during brief nighttime arousals.

CHAPTER 4

A Schedule Emerges
(12–20 Weeks and Beyond)

While you are slogging through the first 3 months of parenthood, time seems to slow down, and you wonder if you will ever find some regularity. Getting through the day is exhausting with a newborn, but then you look up and weeks have flown by.

You have undoubtedly heard about the benefits of getting your baby on a schedule. Despite your best efforts—and possibly self-criticism—the magical schedule might not have taken shape in the first 3 months. But as your baby approaches the 12-week mark, you can likely start to understand how a schedule could be possible. Things start to settle down a lot.

The biggest relief at this age is the winding down of the nightly fussiness or colic. That developmental phase simply passes. Three-month-olds are noticeably less agitated than they were just a few weeks before. It is easier to figure out what they want or need, and they are more easily settled. They are also learning to self-soothe.

But what if your baby is still fussy? Chances are, your baby is simply overtired. It's easy to miss the transition out of the expected fussiness of the first 3 months, especially if your baby is colicky. You have been doing a gymnastics routine to keep your baby calm and (one hopes) get him to sleep. And, like a baseball player at the plate, you will keep repeating whatever has worked even if there is no obvious connection to hitting a home run (good sleep). As the weeks go by, you might notice that your usual heroic efforts—those involving a lot of stimulation, bouncing, or vibrating—are less helpful. That's because your baby has aged out of those strategies and is ready to learn to self-soothe.

Babies are much more aware of their environment at this age, and they are much more aware of *you*. All that soothing can backfire, stimulating your baby instead of lulling her to sleep. Your baby has a harder time falling asleep in your arms, and you have a harder time transferring her to the cot without waking her. It is time for your baby to learn how to fall asleep in the cot. This is the first step toward sleeping through the night. A baby who falls asleep in your arms will need your help to return to sleep when she wakes up during the night. She does not know *how* to fall asleep in the cot. Teaching your baby to fall asleep in the cot at bedtime will make it easier for her to self-soothe during the night and sleep longer without your help.

Your baby might already be falling asleep in the cot some or most of the time. If not, it's time to work on independent sleep more aggressively.

Toning Down the Soothing

Get ready to deflate, or at least repurpose, your exercise ball. The days of endless bouncing are winding down. Keep in mind that an overtired baby has a much harder time self-soothing and being soothed. Catching your baby before she is overtired will make it much easier to phase out the vigorous soothing.

Your already established nap time and bedtime routines will help. For example: the bedtime routine might involve going into the bedroom, making it dark, turning on music, breast- or bottle feeding, reading a book, and then bouncing to sleep. Your baby already has a fairly elaborate set of sleep cues, so you can gradually phase out the more stimulating part. You can slow down your bouncing and then switch to rocking. It might take longer at first, but you can teach your child to respond to this new cue. Keep in mind that you should be using the least stimulating strategy that is necessary to soothe your child.

While you're at it, start working on teaching your baby to fall asleep in the cot. Once he is able to fall asleep without vigorous movement, you can start putting him in the cot drowsy but awake. You can continue to soothe him in the cot by patting, shushing, singing, or rubbing his head or belly. If your baby struggles to fall asleep this way, try avoiding eye contact or even ducking down so that the baby can feel your touch but can't see you. Sometimes babies can't let go and fall asleep if you're engaged. Once he is used to falling asleep in the cot, stop your soothing before he is asleep so that he can learn to do it himself.

If that type of soothing doesn't help, you can say good night and leave the room, allowing him some time to fuss and self-soothe. If he doesn't fall asleep, you can go back in after several minutes to help him settle down. At that point, you can soothe him to sleep and just try again next time or put him back in the cot right away for another try. If you find that your baby does not fall asleep independently after a few days of trying, this method is not for you. Your baby might need to cry to sleep to learn how to self-soothe. The next chapter will take you through the cry-it-out process.

> The process of teaching your baby to fall asleep independently by gradually lessening your soothing is called *fading*.

Keep in mind that this is a fairly loose process designed to see whether your baby is able to gradually learn to fall asleep on his own. This isn't going to create bad habits if done for a short period of time. Your baby already expects you to respond when he cries, so nothing is lost by allowing him some time to settle himself and then responding if he doesn't manage to do it. However—and this is really important—once you use cry-it-out, you should not go back to this kind of routine. Your baby will quickly catch on, and the hard-won sleep training will all slip away.

The Schedule Develops

Some parents are desperate for a schedule, whereas others don't want to feel constrained. But like it or not, the reason your baby needs a schedule is biological. As her body begins to produce melatonin and the cortisol system develops, the natural biorhythm takes over. The biorhythm regulates the sleep/wake cycle, causing her body to slow down for sleep at specific times during the day. We all get our best-quality sleep when we follow our natural biorhythm instead of sleeping at other times. That is why people who work at night and sleep during the day do not feel as refreshed even when they get the same amount of sleep as those with more typical schedules.

When your baby sleeps in sync with her body's natural timing, it is easier for her to get the quantity and quality of sleep she needs. The body simply works best when there is a predictable pattern. However, an overly rigid schedule can be a burden and make you anxious when you can't stick to it. The schedule I recommend does not require military-type precision. Some days your baby won't be ready or won't be able to nap exactly on time. Other days, she'll be tired before the expected time. Allowing yourself some flexibility while sticking with an overall general schedule is usually enough structure to get your baby her best sleep.

> By schedule, I mean a general window of time, essentially plus or minus 30 minutes.

Fortunately, when babies are well rested, the schedule tends to emerge naturally. Following your baby's drowsiness cues and keeping her well rested (as much as possible) will allow the schedule to form when your baby's body is ready. This generally starts around 12 weeks.

Your baby's melatonin system is beginning to establish a more consistent biorhythm as well. The morning nap tends to develop first. You might start to notice that you can count on a nap of an hour or more around 8 or

9 a.m. If your baby is up for the day around 6 a.m., he might take a short nap first and then take the "real" morning nap in the 9 a.m. range.

As the weeks carry on, the second nap will develop and settle around noon. If your baby takes her morning nap closer to 8 a.m. than 9 a.m., the second nap might end up a bit earlier. If she takes a long morning nap, the second nap might be closer to 1 p.m.

As these naps are developing, your baby will take at least one but probably two more naps in the afternoon. Once the first two naps are well settled, the afternoon naps consolidate into one, and you'll have the three-nap schedule. By the time your baby is 4–5 months old, a typical schedule approximates the following:

- 6–7 a.m.: waking up for the day
- 8:30–9:30 a.m.: first nap of the day lasting 1–2 hours (or more). Let your baby sleep as long as he wants.
- 11:30 a.m.–12:30 p.m.: second nap of the day lasting 1–2 hours (or more). Again, let your baby sleep as long as he wants.
- 3:30–4:30 p.m.: Third nap of the day, typically shorter than the other two. Make sure your baby is awake by 5:15 p.m.
- 6–7:30 p.m.: bedtime

During weeks 12–16, continue following drowsiness cues to time the naps. In most cases, the drowsiness cues will coordinate with the baby's natural biorhythm as it develops. The process is often gradual and organic. If naps feel random or chaotic beyond roughly 16 weeks, it's worth it to try to shape the schedule (see Chapter 6).

Why So Much Focus on Naps?

Remember that babies' sleep is a 24-hour cycle. A baby who is overtired during the day is likely to have trouble sleeping well at night and vice versa. Your baby is growing and developing at lightning speed, and she needs sleep to restore her body throughout the day.

Your baby will nap best at home, in the dark, in a cot. She might need some help learning to do that, but the quality of those naps will be best. If your baby hasn't learned to nap in the cot, now is the time. **Napping in the car, stroller, or swing can prevent your baby's brain from settling into the deep, restorative sleep that she needs.** Light and noise will disrupt that process as well. Your baby might nap for just 45 minutes at home, but the quality is better. And if you consistently have her nap at home, she'll start to sleep longer.

A 3-hour nap in the baby carrier or
sling is not likely to be as restorative
as a 3-hour or even a 90-minute nap
at home.

The morning nap is the easiest one to work with because your baby is most rested from the night. Watch your baby for drowsiness cues around 8 or 9 a.m., depending on when he woke up for the day and what kind of night he had. He will probably go down for the nap a little earlier than he usually does in the stroller. The stroller might lull him to sleep even if he's overtired, but he will have an easier time at home if you catch him earlier.

If you're afraid to rock the boat, you're not alone. It's hard to change something that doesn't seem to be broken. But take a step back and look at your situation. Is it feasible to continue doing what you're doing long term? What happens when it rains? Can you really sit in your car for three naps a day? It doesn't get any easier to make these changes. The time is now.

If you want to work gradually, you can change one thing at a time. Switch from the carrier to the stroller first so you can continue to help your baby sleep with motion while she gets used to sleeping someplace other than *on your body*. Next, you might want to continue using the stroller but park it in your baby's room for the nap. Or you can start by putting her in the cot asleep. Then, when your baby is used to that change, work on putting her in the cot slightly awake and patting her or shushing until she is asleep. If she wakes up after a short nap (less than an hour), try to soothe her back to sleep. You can also let her fuss or cry for 10–15 minutes to see if she can go back to sleep on her own.

If the gradual transition doesn't work for you or your baby, you might need to use a cry-it-out strategy (see Chapter 6).

It's impossible to stay home for every nap. Napping at home should be the norm, but your baby will have to be more flexible sometimes. A trip to the doctor shouldn't induce panic just because it coincides with nap time. Some babies nap better than others when they are on the go. Once your baby is napping well, you will get a better sense of how much you can push her. Here are a few rules of thumb:

- Try to have the first nap at home. It's the most important, and it gets the day started on the right track.
- If you have a choice, sacrifice the third nap. The quality of the late-afternoon ("disco") nap is not as critical. Its purpose is to take the edge off of the afternoon so your baby isn't overtired at bedtime. If

that nap happens in the stroller or carrier, it's less likely to disrupt things.

- Don't push your baby too much at one time. Try not to do consecutive naps on the go. If you do have to be out all day, plan the next day to be quieter and closer to home.

The Early Bedtime

When parents come to me for help, the first thing I look for is a bedtime that is too late. When babies (and kids) go to bed too late, the whole night is affected. Bedtimes get drawn out with protest, difficulty soothing/settling, and—later— separation anxiety. Night waking multiplies and becomes harder to manage, particularly around 4 a.m. Early waking also sets in, throwing the entire day's schedule off kilter. It is hard to imagine that a late bedtime wreaks silent havoc until 4 a.m., but it's true. Fortunately, adjusting the bedtime is straightforward and usually works quickly.

Why is the early bedtime so important? It all comes back to adrenaline. If babies go to bed overtired, the night is likely to suffer. Adrenaline makes it harder for babies to fall asleep, sleep deeply, and return to sleep during normal nighttime arousals. The infant body clock is set to a bedtime between 6:30 and 7:30 p.m. Remember, babies have melatonin levels higher than those of adults, and those levels build up in the afternoon and evening. As the night wears on, the body needs more and more help to stay awake, and that comes in the form of adrenaline.

For the first 3 months, "bedtime" was probably an arbitrary decision based on the frequent feeding schedule and the 90-minute rule. Babies start to get a longer stretch of sleep at night, typically starting around 10 p.m. But as the body clock settles, the melatonin kicks in earlier and the bedtime must move. That tends to happen around 10–14 weeks.

The shift to an earlier bedtime could occur without much effort: your baby might go down for a nap at 7:30 p.m. and sleep until midnight. But if it doesn't happen on its own, it's up to you to make the shift. If 10 p.m. is the average bedtime, start the bedtime routine before the last evening nap instead of after it. Your baby will start responding to the bedtime cues as they happen in sync with his body clock. Initially, your baby might still wake up after a couple of hours even with the early bedtime. The difference is that you will not get him up or interact with him in a stimulating way. Keep the lights low. Take care of business. Get him back to bed.

Louise: The Early Bedtime Works Wonders

Louise was 10 weeks old when her mother asked for my advice. She was still waking multiple times per night and not on a predictable schedule. When we discussed the schedule, it was clear that it was time to start putting Louise to bed earlier. Although she was sleeping in a swing or car seat during the early part of the evening, that last "nap" was in the middle of the action while her parents made dinner and watched television. They were doing the bedtime routine around 10 p.m. and putting her in the cot for the night.

Louise's parents had begun to notice that the evening nap was getting tricky. Sometimes she would fight it. Sometimes she would be extremely fussy, and it would take heroic soothing (or extended feeding) to get her to settle. Sometimes she'd sleep for 20 minutes and pop awake, repeating the cycle and getting more and more exhausted as the evening wore on.

Based on my advice, Louise's parents moved the bedtime routine to 7 p.m. and started putting her down in the cot between 7:15 and 7:30. Within a few days, the night waking reduced to two feedings. Over the next couple of weeks, Louise began waking just once and eventually began sleeping through the night.

In general, the effect of bedtime overfatigue accumulates over time. That means you might not have a problem at first, but it will sneak up on you in the end. Night waking worsens. Early waking gets earlier. And it's easy to overlook the culprit because the problems emerge gradually. But if bedtime is later than 7:30 p.m. and your baby struggles to fall asleep, wakes up during the night, or wakes up before 6 a.m. on a regular basis, try moving the bedtime earlier for a week.

I know that an early bedtime is a drag. It might seem impossible. Parents who work outside the home will have limited—if any—time with the baby at night. I did the day-care dash myself, with each of my two kids: rushing to leave work on time, picking them up at day care, running home, and working nonstop to get through dinner and a (necessarily brief) bedtime routine. If we were lucky, my husband would get home in time to put the baby to bed. Many nights, he just couldn't get home in time.

It's hard. It feels like you are depriving your child. But really, you are the one who will feel deprived. Of course your baby needs to spend time with you, but in the hierarchy of needs at 7 p.m. on a weeknight, your baby needs to sleep. We all feel guilty when we don't spend "enough" time with our kids. But we shouldn't make up for it by causing sleep deprivation.

Although you do need time with your baby, you also need your family to function in a sustainable way. That means everyone sleeping through the night. The trade-off

Can't my baby sleep from 9 p.m. to 9 a.m. instead of 7 to 7? The short answer is: probably not. **The vast majority of babies get a surge of melatonin early in the evening, so putting them to bed later will not lead to more sleep.** Chances are, your baby will still wake up at the same time—or earlier—even if she goes to bed later. That sleep deficit will accumulate and lead to night waking, short naps, and a whole lot of crankiness.

for spending time with your baby when she should be sleeping is that you will be seeing a lot more of your baby when *you* should be sleeping. That's unsustainable, and there's really no reason it should be the case.

So how will you make this work? First, don't panic. Figure out a short-term plan, maybe a week or two, for getting your baby to bed on time consistently. Once you determine your baby's window of bedtime, a rhythm will emerge. The early bedtime leads to better night sleep. Better night sleep helps naps to lengthen and consolidate, keeping your baby in a predictable rhythm of good sleep. You'll start to think more clearly because you will be more rested. Then you can think about a longer-term plan for getting your baby the sleep she needs.

The Schedule Evolves

As your baby gets older, the schedule will evolve. Naps lengthen and spread out. Your baby is able to stay up longer between naps. And the bedtime might push to the later end of the bedtime window. Next, your baby will drop a nap from the schedule, and the bedtime will have to move earlier. Here's what to look for:

3–5 months: The three-nap schedule emerges, and the bedtime moves earlier.

6–8 or 9 months: The first two naps might lengthen and spread out. The third nap starts to be less reliable. The bedtime moves earlier on days when the third nap doesn't happen.

8–10 months: The third nap disappears, and bedtime moves earlier. Naps typically start between 9 and 10 a.m. and between 1:00 and 2:00 p.m. If the first two naps remain earlier in the day, gradually extend the amount of time between them, watching to make sure that the length of the nap does not shorten. Move the nap 15 minutes later every 1–2 days. If the nap length shortens, your baby is getting too tired before the second nap. You will have to work even more slowly to push the nap later. Wait several days—until the nap length stabilizes—before moving.

I get a lot of calls about the so-called 8-month regression, when babies who were sleeping through the night start waking up again, usually around

> As a general rule, 6 p.m. is the earliest bedtime I recommend. Although some babies can sleep more than 12 hours at night, most do not. If you put your baby down before 6 p.m., he could easily wake for the day before 6 a.m., which creates problems for naps. However, there are times when a baby can really benefit from a very early bedtime. If your baby is a mess, you can put him down at 5:30. If the next day starts too early, you will know that it's better to stick to 6 p.m.

4 a.m. The answer almost always lies with the bedtime. The third nap has dropped out, but the bedtime has not moved earlier to compensate. A simple bedtime adjustment is usually all it takes to get back on track.

Always keep your eye on the interval between the last nap and bedtime. When your baby first drops the third nap, that interval is likely to be too long. Temporarily moving the bedtime earlier will smooth out the adjustment to the new daytime schedule. As the naps settle, the bedtime will push later again.

10–15 months: Most babies remain on a two-nap schedule with naps at 9 or 10 a.m. and 1:30–2:30 p.m. until they reach 14–18 months. The bedtime gradually pushes to the later end of the window, around 7:30. But 8 p.m. is still too late.

14–18 months: The second nap drops away during this period. You might notice that your baby doesn't fall asleep for the first nap. Or the first nap is starting later (10–10:30 a.m.) and lasting 2–3 hours. Even though there is time for a second nap, your baby doesn't fall asleep. You are now down to one nap. Once again, move the bedtime earlier as your baby adjusts to this schedule. Once she is settled into a nice (preferably 2–3 hours long) midday nap, the bedtime will push later again.

If your baby is struggling with a single nap that ends too early, gradually push the start time later in increments of 15–20 minutes every few days. Once the nap is happening around 11–11:30 a.m., you might stick with that nap time until your baby seems to be able to stay up longer in the morning. You'll notice less crankiness and frustration in the late morning. That will indicate that you can push the nap to noon or 12:30 p.m. You'll maintain this schedule more or less until your baby (now your toddler) drops the nap entirely sometime between ages 2½ and 5 years.

What If You Don't Have a Choice About Nap Times?

Sometimes the schedule isn't under your control. Some day-care centers have specific nap times that might not be perfectly aligned with your baby's developmental stage. Nanny shares have to coordinate with other babies' needs. And preschool or activity schedules don't always coincide with age-appropriate nap schedules.

Obviously, when you can, you should choose activities that don't regularly interfere with your child's naps and child-care providers who won't force your child into a schedule he's not ready for. If your baby must drop a nap prematurely, be prepared to compensate with an early bedtime. In most cases, it is best to stick with the same nap schedule on weekends. However, if your baby is really struggling with the transition, reverting to the old schedule on weekends can be a stopgap solution to keep him rested while his body adjusts.

Key Points from Chapter 4

- By 12 weeks, your baby's body clock is settling into a rhythm.
- Naps will lengthen and become more reliable, settling into a three-nap schedule.
- The early bedtime is essential for lengthening night sleep.
- Stimulating forms of soothing—bouncing, rocking, pacing the floor—become less effective. Your baby must learn to soothe himself because you are too distracting.
- After the 3-month mark, it becomes harder for your baby to fall asleep in your arms and *much* harder to transfer him into the cot asleep. At this point, falling asleep in the cot is key.
- Phasing out the extreme soothing and fostering more self-soothing will help your baby to self-soothe in the night instead of waking up seeking comfort from you.

CHAPTER 5

Sleeping Through the Night

Every new mum has a friend whose child spontaneously started sleeping through the night at 6 weeks old. Do yourself a favor: don't compare notes. Maybe that friend can be helpful, but she's had it easy. Her advice might not apply to your situation. And comparisons could undermine your confidence in your own parenting, something you can't afford right now. If you're not as lucky as your friend, you're going to need to help your child learn to sleep.

Again: A well-rested child will gradually start to sleep for longer and

> Sleep is not just about nighttime. It is a 24-hour process, and when it doesn't go well, it is a 24-hour problem. When parents come to me with a problem sleeper, I look at the entire day and night to find an entry point to break into the cycle and reroute the sleep onto the right track.

longer stretches. And some babies gradually start to sleep through the night on their own. But most babies need help learning how to soothe themselves and fall asleep. People may tell you to put your child down awake and leave the room. If that feels cruel and impossible to carry out, you can work through this process more gradually.

Step 1: Get Your Baby as Rested as Possible

Much of night waking is caused by overfatigue. Remember that babies who are overtired will fight sleep at bedtime and wake up more frequently, all because of the adrenaline in their systems.

- Your baby should have a consistent early bedtime between 6 and 8 p.m. That means starting the routine early enough to have your baby in bed at the appropriate time. Most babies between the ages of 8 weeks and 2 years have a natural bedtime of 6:30–7:30 p.m. If your baby is very overtired, consider making the bedtime 6:00. Your child's drowsiness signs will indicate when the time is right. If you miss the window of opportunity (i.e., there is lots of crying or your baby resists sleep), start the bedtime routine earlier the following night.

• Your baby should have an age-appropriate nap schedule (see Chapter 4) and nap at home or at day care most of the time. Depending on your baby's age, she will take one to three naps (even more if she is very overtired or very young). Napping in a cot gives your baby the best possible circumstances for restorative sleep and creates strong sleep associations that help with self-soothing. Your baby will come to expect the routine and respond to it consistently.

Step 2: Create Sleep Cues and Stop Feeding to Sleep

• Your bedtime routine transitions your baby from active play to sleep by establishing sleep cues. This teaches your baby what to expect and sends a clear message that playtime is over. Sleep associations help your baby to relax as the routine winds down. Chapter 2 includes details about how to do this.

• Most of the time, your baby should fall asleep *after* feeding, not *while* feeding. Your baby might still fall asleep in your arms at this stage, but she should not fall asleep on the breast or bottle.

Babies who fall asleep while feeding will develop a very strong feeding/sleep association. When they wake up throughout the night—a normal function of the sleep cycle—they will have difficulty returning to sleep without sucking or feeding. If your baby consistently falls asleep while feeding, start the bedtime routine earlier and add a sleep cue (a book, snuggle, or song) between feeding and sleep.

• Establish methods of soothing your baby without feeding. Breaking the feeding/sleep association is hardest. When you are able to soothe your baby by rocking, shushing, patting, singing, etc., your baby will more easily transition to self-soothing.

Step 3: Teach Your Baby to Fall Asleep in the Cot

This is important because your baby will be waking up and falling asleep multiple times during the night. If your baby needs to fall asleep in your arms at bedtime, she will need you to repeat that process during the night. Another important reason your baby should fall asleep in the cot is that you become more and more stimulating as your baby gets older. Your baby is soothed by you but also wants to play with you.

After all, you probably can't fall
asleep with someone staring at you.
The same becomes true for your
baby as she gets older.

The fastest, most reliable way to teach your baby to fall asleep in the cot is by letting her cry. You can skip ahead to that method (Step 8) if you are ready. If not, work on getting your baby to fall asleep in the cot gradually.

- Start by putting your baby in the cot almost asleep and doing whatever is necessary to help him fall asleep outside of your arms. This could be patting, shushing, singing, or keeping your hand on him. Avoid making eye contact or engaging him. Your baby will probably protest this change. If necessary, pick him up, calm him down, and put him back down in the cot to try again. **NOTE: If you are already using the cry-it-out method, do not revert to this kind of soothing.**
- Over several days or weeks, as your baby responds to your soothing, gradually lessen your efforts. For example, keep your hand on him instead of patting; stay quiet instead of singing. As you do this, begin to stop the soothing process before your baby

falls asleep fully. This way, you are gradually teaching your baby to fall asleep on his own.

It is important to note that not all babies respond well to gradual strategies. If your baby keeps up a forceful protest for many nights, it makes sense to consider using that crying for learning purposes (i.e., cry-it-out).

Step 4: Figure Out Why Your Baby Is Still Waking Up

If your baby is reasonably well rested but still requires attention during the night, it is either true hunger requiring your response (this happens with younger babies) or the waking is simply reinforced by your soothing and attention. Your baby is used to waking up and getting lots of warmth, food, and attention. This encourages her to keep waking up, even after she is capable of getting all of her nutrition during the day. Over time, that attention becomes so stimulating that your baby will have a hard time going back to sleep. Your doctor will be able to tell you whether your baby is gaining weight well enough to make it through the night without feedings. Once that is the case, your baby can learn to make it through the night emotionally as well.

Need Versus Want

Parents often struggle at this point because they don't want to deny their babies the attention they are seeking. This is where it is very important to remember that while your baby might *want* you, she does not physiologically *need* you. What she needs—to grow, to learn, to be happy and cheerful—is sleep. Your presence becomes a distraction. Often babies become more agitated when parents respond to them in the night. It is as if they are angry that the parent is unable to soothe them. They want the soothing, yet it doesn't help. And even if it does help settle the baby, it can serve to reinforce the waking and deprive the baby of sleep over the course of the night. If she learns to get back to sleep independently, she will eventually stop waking up so much.

As parents, we are constantly weighing what is best for our children. And though we hate to break it to them, often what is best for them is not what they want. They want to poke their fingers in electrical sockets, eat dirt, and pull dogs' tails. They want to stay home from school, hoard toys from their friends and siblings, or eat a diet consisting exclusively of cheese. Our judgment as parents is needed to guide our children toward the things they need. Even more than vegetables, children need sleep.

(And the more rested they are, the more amenable they are to trying new things—like vegetables.) Providing structure and guidelines is not "laying down the law" in an insensitive, authoritarian way. *It is simply taking care of your child.*

Step 5: Pick a Strategy: Methodical Step-by-Step or Cut to the Chase

At this point, you need to sit down with your partner and discuss your plan of action for sleep. You are a team, and you will need to be ready to support each other. Discuss and address your concerns in advance so you'll know what to do when things get challenging. You won't be able to think clearly at 3 a.m. when your baby starts to cry. Having a plan in place will help you to remain consistent when all you want to do is throw in the towel.

> This is not the time to be wishy-washy. You must have a plan, and you both must commit to it.

My advice in most cases is to cut to the chase. Letting your baby cry is really hard, but so is working slowly and methodically. It is hard to keep pushing ahead when each step requires resolve. It takes longer, so it requires more discipline and perseverance. And it doesn't necessarily involve less crying. If you add up all the crying over the weeks that it takes to work through the gradual methods, you will have many more tears than if you skipped right to letting your baby cry.

That said, I can understand the motivation to work gradually, and I have helped countless families through the process. If you don't think you'll be able to stick with letting your baby cry, don't start. It is worse to start and quit. Gradual methods *can* work.

Step 6: Weaning from Night Feedings

Your doctor says your baby does not need night feedings, but you are still breast- or bottlefeeding your baby multiple times per night. Those feedings are most likely serving to comfort or soothe rather than nourish your baby. Even if your baby is still taking in 30–40 ml per waking, she will quickly start to eat more during the day when you cut out the night feedings. Weaning the baby from night feedings will help her start sleeping through the night. If she does not start sleeping through the night after being weaned, you will at least be confident that she isn't hungry.

Newborns need to feed around the clock, of course. Their stomachs are tiny, their jaws are weak, and they are growing exponentially. But as they grow, they start to be able to feed more efficiently, taking in what they need more quickly and in fewer feedings. Sometime around 12 weeks, often sooner and depending on weight, babies are able to take in 24 hours' worth of calories in 12 *daytime* hours. At this point, they can and should learn to sleep without feeding.

Eliminating night feeding when the baby is physiologically capable of feeding enough during the day allows the body's digestion to slow down during the night. Your baby does not have to be full at all times to sleep. In fact, a baby will sleep more deeply if the metabolism stays steadily slow during the night.

Options for Night Weaning

- *If you are breastfeeding, gradually decrease the amount of time the baby spends at the breast.* A good rule of thumb is to cut the amount of time in half for each feeding every 1–2 days. This requires that you remain alert in the middle of the night and watch the clock. When you reach the end of the allotted time, remove the baby from your breast and soothe with other methods. If possible, put him back down drowsy but awake.
- *Bottle-feed at night (expressed milk or formula).* This makes it much easier to decrease the amount of milk/formula that the baby takes in at each feed-

ing. Decrease by 30 ml at each feeding each night. If the bottle is the only way to soothe your baby, ask your doctor whether you can switch to water once you have weaned your baby from milk.

- *Have your partner bottle-feed at night.* Decrease the amount of milk or formula as described above. **Babies often protest when the breastfeeding mother tries to bottle-feed.**

Maggie: Using the Bottle to Night-Wean

Maggie was almost 6 months old when her parents contacted me. She was waking five to six times during the night and feeding back to sleep. Often, though, she would become overstimulated, and it would take her a long time and lots of comfort feeding to settle back down. Her parents were reluctant to let her cry it out, but they were both exhausted. We agreed to first try to night-wean Maggie. Her mother attempted to space out the feedings during the night, but Maggie protested so much that her mother gave up. Although Maggie was not fond of the bottle, it seemed like the best option to move things along.

Maggie's father took over night duty and gave her the bottle at each night waking. She was not happy about this change and she took only 30 ml of milk on the first night. She rejected the bottle entirely on the second night and never resumed night feeding. Her night waking reduced to an average of three times per night. That was quite an improvement for her but not enough to get her the rest she needed. Later in this chapter, you will hear how Maggie's parents taught her to sleep through the night.

Step 7: Weaning from Night Soothing

Babies need to learn to soothe themselves back to sleep. This is not a skill that magically develops. Many parents want to try gradual methods to help their babies sleep through the night. These methods tend to take longer than so-called extinction methods, and they require tremendous consistency. There is one major caveat here: if your efforts to soothe backfire and your baby becomes more agitated, you will be better off skipping to the cry-it-out methods below. Here are some options for weaning from night soothing:

- *Delegate*: Have the non-breastfeeding partner take over night soothing. Breastfeeding mothers often have a difficult time soothing without feeding because the smell of milk and the strong feeding association frustrate the baby. Having the other parent take over night soothing can help. Sometimes, if the baby doesn't get what she wants (MAMA!), she will learn that it is not worth it to wake up. This does *not* mean that the baby likes the other parent less. It is simply that your baby has learned to expect certain forms of soothing. Changing the routine can "loosen" that association and help her learn to self-soothe more effectively.

- *Gradually withdraw the soothing*: Follow this progression, moving one step after 1–2 days of success.
  - ◗ Soothe the baby by picking him up but not feeding him. Put him back in the cot asleep.
  - ◗ Pick up the baby (but do not feed him), soothe, and put him back down slightly awake. Continue soothing him in the cot by patting, shushing, rubbing his head, singing, or humming.
  - ◗ Soothe the baby in the cot until he is asleep, without picking him up.
  - ◗ Soothe the baby in the cot without picking him up, until he is calm but not fully asleep.

Step 8: The Final Hurdle: Cry-It-Out

Some babies respond to gentle methods and start sleeping through the night. However, it is no failure of parenting if your baby needs more help. Most babies require some guidance, whether it is falling asleep for the night or getting back to sleep independently when they wake up in the night.

As babies get older, they start to fight sleep to be with

you. They also start to learn cause and effect (e.g., I cry → I get soothed). As long as you continue to soothe your baby in the middle of the night, you can expect your baby to wake up to be with you. When you stop soothing, your baby will learn to do it herself. Sometimes this can be done gradually, as described in the "Weaning from Night Soothing" section. But sometimes efforts to soothe become more agitating for the baby. If that happens, your baby is essentially telling you that she needs you to leave her alone.

Timing

If your baby is 3–4 months old and healthy, she should be able to learn to self-soothe. Babies can often learn to self-soothe much earlier, but you should consult your GP or health visitor to determine whether your child is ready.

Some books suggest waiting until the baby is 6 months old. But unless there are competing concerns (feeding problems, slow weight gain, medical issues), I recommend using cry-it-out methods during the 3- to 4-month window if possible. And, from a practical standpoint, the sooner your family is sleeping, the better. However, if your baby is more than 4 months old already, you have not missed your chance. You have probably realized that your baby's sleep isn't magically improving, so it's time for you to find a solution.

Babies begin to develop separation anxiety as they reach 6 months of age, and the sleep-training process tends to go more smoothly before that time.

Extinction Explained

The technical term for cry-it-out methods is *extinction*. The terminology might sound draconian, but extinction methods are called this because they "extinguish" the baby's learned association between crying and being tended to in the night.

I want to be clear: extinction methods involve crying. Letting your baby cry goes against every instinct in a parent's body. Your baby's cry is pitched to mobilize you. And leaving your baby alone involves inhibiting one of nature's most powerful instincts. Most parents naturally ask why they should ignore these instincts. Put simply, it is because there is a difference between a cry of desire and a cry of necessity, between a cry of protest and

Infants learn early on that crying produces soothing, feeding, and attention at night. This happens through a process called **operant conditioning**. When a behavior (waking or crying) is reinforced with a reward (food), it is more likely to occur in the future. Removing the reward ends the reinforcement. Initially the baby will stick to what worked in the past (waking and crying). But with time, the lack of reward will teach the baby to stop waking and crying out of habit. The process of removing rewards to eliminate a behavior is called **extinction**.

a cry of distress, even though most parents have difficulty distinguishing the difference at first.

Letting your baby cry when he should be sleeping teaches him to sleep when his body is tired. It teaches him to return to sleep quickly and seamlessly during normal nighttime arousals. It teaches him to get down to the business of sleep. Babies who learn to sleep will start to tell you when they want to go to bed, and they will even get mad when you keep them up too late.

Preparation and Safety

- Your baby should be in a separate room when you use extinction methods. If you share a room with your baby, sleep in another room or area while you are using these methods. Plan to sleep away from your baby until he is reliably sleeping through the night for at least 1 week.
- Your baby should not be able to see you or sense your presence. (No sleeping on the floor under the cot!) **Your nonresponsive presence is more upsetting to your child than your absence.**
- Before you start, make sure that you will be able to keep a consistent schedule for 2 weeks. That means reasonably consistent bedtimes and naps and avoiding travel. Most babies respond more quickly than

2 weeks, but it is important to be prepared for an extended process if necessary.

- Assess your baby's cot for SIDS safety.
- Lower the cot mattress; babies often hit milestones (rolling over, sitting, standing) during this process. Lowering the mattress will ensure that your baby is safe in the cot.
- Do not swaddle the baby while sleep training. Your baby will start to roll sooner or later and will need the use of his arms. He will also use his hands to self-soothe.

The Process

- Perform your usual bedtime routine, but stop soothing before the baby is asleep.
- If your baby is not settling down, do not spend extra time trying to calm him. He will probably become agitated again when you put him in the cot awake, so it's better to just forge ahead.
- Put your baby in the cot awake at his normal bedtime. Some books recommend using a later bedtime so the baby will be extra tired. I prefer to use the early bedtime in an effort to put the baby to bed before she is overtired, so her body won't be fighting sleep.

- Let your baby cry to fall asleep at bedtime and for each night waking until morning. (If you must keep a feeding, see below.)
- If you respond sometimes but not others, your baby will cry harder and longer, trying to crack your code and elicit the response.

You must be consistent. Babies do not understand ambiguity.

Jackie: The Case for Consistency All Night Long

Jackie was 3 months old when her parents contacted me. They were at their wits' end. Jackie had reflux, colic, and couldn't self-soothe. Prior to contacting me, her parents had been sleep training with cry-it-out for 2 weeks, but she was still crying for an extended period at bedtime and waking multiple times during the night.

It turned out that Jackie's parents had decided to use cry-it-out at bedtime to teach her to fall asleep, but they continued to respond to her night waking, feeding on demand, and soothing her back to sleep. Although they had some initial progress, within a few days Jackie figured out the terms and started waking up as soon as 40 minutes after falling asleep at bedtime. All of the attention she was getting during the night had caused her sleep to fragment more.

Jackie's parents opted to keep one feeding as an interim

step because they were uncomfortable dropping all night feeding at once. They ignored all crying until midnight, fed once, and then did not respond again until 6 a.m. Jackie improved dramatically, and they dropped the night feeding altogether.

Crying with Checks: AKA the "Ferber Method"

This method, developed by Dr. Richard Ferber, involves leaving your baby alone to cry for increasing intervals of time. After the allotted time, one parent goes into the baby's room and soothes verbally for 1–3 minutes. The parent must leave the room regardless of whether the baby is still crying. The process below is repeated each time the baby wakes during the night.

- *Night 1:* Let the baby cry for 5 minutes before checking. Then check after 10 minutes, then 15 minutes. Continue checking at 15-minute intervals until the baby is quiet.
- *Night 2:* Intervals are 10, 15, and 20 minutes, with continued checking at 20-minute intervals.
- *Night 3:* Intervals are 15, 20, and 30 minutes, with continued checking at 30-minute intervals.

If you are unable to last for 5 minutes, start with 3, then 5, then 10 minutes on the first night. The most important part of this method is lengthening the amount of time after each check. However, the less you check, the faster the method will work.

You should start this method at bedtime, following your consistent bedtime routine. Letting your baby cry at bedtime often leads to less crying throughout the night. In other words, learning starts immediately. But do not throw in the towel if your baby has an extended bout of crying in the night. Over the course of several days of consistent sleep training, the intensity and duration of crying diminish.

Maggie, Part 2: Learning to Sleep Through the Night

After night weaning Maggie, her parents remained committed to trying to avoid letting her cry it out. She was still waking three times per night, and her father remained on night duty. He worked hard to teach her to fall asleep in the cot, but she became agitated when he would put her in the cot awake and try to soothe her there. Her night waking lengthened as she became overstimulated, and over the course of about a week, everyone lost patience. Maggie had essentially told her parents that it was time to move on to a new strategy.

Maggie's parents felt unable to leave her alone to cry without checking on her, so we agreed that the Ferber method was their best bet. After the first night, Maggie's parents reported that she did not cry as long as they had feared and that it wasn't as hard to hear her cry as they had anticipated. She woke up three times, crying the first time on and off for 1 hour, crying for 10 minutes the second time, and crying on and off from 4 to 6 a.m. Her father reported that she fell asleep much more easily than she did when he had been trying to soothe her. He also decided to wait longer before going in to check, because it seemed easier for Maggie to fall asleep without him going in so much. By the third night, her crying was down to less than 5 minutes, and by the end of the week, she was sleeping through the night.

Crying Without Checks

Checking on your baby can backfire. If your baby becomes more agitated and upset when you check on her, consider letting her cry without checking. The checking itself does not do much for your baby. It functions more to reassure parents that the baby is all right. Extinction methods often work faster without checks.

Checking can also be a problem if you are unable to be consistent with the timing. Having the option of checking can lead parents to cut the crying intervals short, which undermines the process. If you are unable to be consistent, abandon the checks.

The rules for crying without checks (extinction) are extremely simple. Following them is a gut-wrenching challenge but one that pays enormous dividends for your child: At the end of the bedtime routine, put the baby in her cot, say something soothing, and leave the room. Do not open the door until morning.

Helen: How Checking Can Backfire

Helen was 6 months old when her parents contacted me. She was able to go to sleep at night without much fuss, although she was being put into the cot fully or almost fully asleep. Helen would sleep for a few hours and then wake up to feed every 2 hours for the rest of the night.

Helen's parents were reluctant to use cry-it-out without checking because Helen had once suffered a life-threatening allergic reaction. Although that did not happen in the cot when she was unattended, her parents were uncomfortable with the idea of not checking on her during the night.

The problem was that Helen really, really wanted to feed during the night and she was unable to transition through mild arousals back to sleep without it. We started by moving the bedtime from 8 p.m. to 7 p.m. and adjusting nap times to establish a good schedule. Then we switched to bottles during the night instead of breastfeeding. Then we hit a wall.

Helen was having none of it. She was crying and protesting and not learning to sleep. We tried everything we could think of to get her to sleep without feeding, and nothing worked. After 1 week, everyone was more exhausted than when we started.

Our attempts to find a new way out went around in circles. So we began to discuss crying.

Helen's parents were reluctant, but they could now see that the leap from breastfeedng back to sleep to self-soothing was not possible in baby steps. On the first night of cry-it-out, they used timed checks to lessen their anxiety. But Helen quickly put a stop to that. She became so upset when they checked that they stopped going in. By the second night, Helen was waking just once. And by the end of the week, she was sleeping through the night.

Keeping a Scheduled Feeding

Decide before you start whether you will feed your baby during the night or in the very early morning. **Babies often have a strong arousal around 4 a.m.** Some parents choose to feed the baby at that time and plan to work on that waking later. Other parents let the baby cry it out until 6 a.m. from the start.

If your doctor has advised you to keep a night feeding or if you just can't fathom not feeding your baby during the night, you can still use the cry-it-out method to teach your baby to sleep. Set a specific interval after which you will feed, either midway through the night (the first time the baby wakes up after midnight) or the tricky 4 a.m. waking. Let the baby cry at bedtime and every time he wakes *except for* the scheduled feeding time. The feeding should be all business (and by bottle if possible). Avoid long, comfort feedings and put the baby back in the cot as soon as the feeding is finished. Put your baby back into the cot awake and let him cry again. If your baby falls asleep while feeding, there is no need to wake him.

It is important to note that using extinction methods with a feeding can slow down the learning process. Babies learn to fall asleep without crying because each time they wake up, you are consistent in your response (i.e., lack of response). But when you introduce a feeding, it can reset the cry → soothing expectation, and your baby might cry more the next time she wakes. That doesn't mean it's useless to sleep-train with a feeding. It's just important to understand the pros and cons of each approach.

Dream Feeding

The concept of dream feeding is based on the assumption that babies wake up because they are hungry. Dream feeding involves feeding the baby while she is essentially asleep, before she wakes up and demands your attention. In most cases, dream feeding isn't necessary. In rare cases in which the baby has extreme difficulty night weaning, dream feeding can be helpful. But whenever you disrupt a sleeping baby, you run the risk of making things worse. If the baby wakes up completely, she will be at an inopportune place in her sleep cycle and will likely be very difficult to soothe to sleep again.

Dream feeding also keeps the digestive system active through the night. This actually seems to make a baby hungrier during the later part of the night, perhaps because her metabolism has not slowed as it should during sleep. Once your baby is capable of consolidating feeding during the day, night feeding—even dream feeding—encourages unnecessary night waking.

Shane: The Pros and Cons of Dream Feeding

Shane was 12 weeks old when his parents contacted me. Shane had the typical rocky start: reflux, crying, and not much sleep. His mother was also struggling with moderate postnatal depression, which is extremely common in such situations. There was so much crying and so little sleep that Shane's parents decided (with their doctor's approval) to begin using cry-it-out when he was 9 weeks old.

Shane was born on the small side, less than 6 pounds, and although he was growing well, his parents were concerned that he needed at least one night feeding. They began using cry-it-out without feeding but quickly became convinced that Shane really needed to eat. They found that when they responded to Shane's crying with feeding, night waking increased. So they decided to try an 11 p.m. dream feed.

The dream feed worked well: Shane barely roused and slept soundly for several hours. However, he continued to wake up at 4:30 a.m. most nights and cry for 30–60 minutes, sometimes until his parents gave up and started the day. Feeding him at that time resulted in more waking the following night. The crying was very hard to endure, but everyone agreed that the alternatives would jeopardize the gains that Shane had made.

After a couple of weeks, Shane's parents contacted me again as their patience with the 4:30 a.m. waking had worn out. Having been in similar circumstances with other families, I was fairly certain that the dream feed was linked to the night waking. Shane's parents were ready to try to get rid of it. This time, Shane immediately began eating more during the day and began sleeping through the night in a matter of days.

Simplifying the cot cleanup will help you through this process. Regular cot sheets can be impossible to manage, especially under stressful circumstances. Get a few of the sheets that fasten to the cot slats, on top of the regular cot sheet, so you can get the cot cleaned up quickly and get back to sleep training.

Vomit

It's an awful truth, but some babies vomit when they cry hard or for long periods of time. This makes an already difficult process much more painful—for you—and gross. If your baby is prone to vomit, you can start by checking at shorter intervals (3 minutes, then 5, then 10). This might not prevent vomiting, but it can help. If your baby does throw up, clean her up and go back to letting her cry. Vomiting might slow down the learning process, but if you ersevere, your baby should be falling asleep with minimal or no crying (which means no vomiting) soon. Keep in mind that the vomit is caused by a gag reflex and not by the distress itself.

How to Survive Cry-It-Out

There are no two ways about it: letting your baby cry is hard and there is no pleasant way to get through it, but these strategies can help.

- Watch the clock: This is essential because 5 minutes feels like 5 hours. It is also essential to help you track your progress. You will have difficulty remembering the details of this whole process over time (thankfully!), but you will want to have a reasonable sense of how long your baby cried.
- **Do not** watch the baby on a video monitor: If you must, check the monitor at timed intervals; watching continuously will undermine your resolve.
- Distract yourself: Listen to music, watch a movie, play video games.
- Seek support: Call friends and relatives, anyone who is awake and willing to listen without judging.

- Take turns taking breaks: Because you don't yet know how long your baby can cry, the first bout of crying can be the hardest to endure. If you need an escape, go for a walk, go to a bookshop, go to the gym while your partner holds vigil.
- Drown out the crying: Take a shower, put on headphones. Take turns wearing earplugs.
- Clutch each other. Seriously.
- In advance, write down a list of the reasons that you are doing this and read it aloud while your baby cries. Examples include:
  - My baby needs to learn to sleep.
  - My baby is protesting. She doesn't really need me.
  - If I tried to soothe her, it would upset her more.
  - I am doing this *for* my baby, not *to* my baby.
  - She will eventually fall asleep.
  - If I give in now, it will be much harder later.

Your Baby's Reaction

Some babies wake up all smiles after the first night of sleep training. Others, typically older babies, take some time to adjust. They might be clingy initially. They also might start to cry when they see the cot. This is normal and temporary. It does not represent a breach of the parental bond, nor does it mean that you have made your child hate the cot. This is a learning process that is difficult for some for the first few days. If you remain consistent and keep going, your child will be well rested and happy. Keep up a positive front. Give your baby lots of affection, but don't send the message that something is wrong. For a longer discussion of the effects of extinction methods, see Appendix A.

How Long Does It Take?

Unfortunately, there are no guarantees about how long this will take. Most babies respond within a few days (some in just one day), particularly if there is no checking. Typically, there is a lot of crying the first night. The second night is sometimes better, but sometimes worse as babies make one last-ditch effort to summon you. The third night is typically much better, and things continue to improve. However, progress is not always linear. Think of it as a zigzag line that moves in an upward direction. Some babies take longer to adjust.

Does It Last?

Yes, it does. But that doesn't mean you'll never have to let your baby cry again. When your baby is sick, you will tend to her. Once she gets well, she might have become very comfortable with your nighttime attention. Other blips may occur when you're traveling, moving, or changing day cares or babysitters, or on special occasions when the schedule goes out the window. But you won't be starting from scratch. Babies remember what it's like to get good sleep, and they rebound quickly when you help them.

Key Points from Chapter 5

- Some babies just don't transition smoothly to falling asleep in the cot and sleeping through the night no matter how diligent and devoted their parents are along the way.
- Allowing your baby to cry to sleep teaches him how to fall asleep independently.
- Crying it out also breaks the cycle of night waking, which is no longer a biological necessity but a habit reinforced every time you appear to help.
- This process is emotionally challenging for most parents, but it is safe, effective, and—in most cases—fast.
- By teaching your baby to get the sleep that she needs, you are providing her with an essential skill that she will rely upon—and thank you for—for the rest of her life.

CHAPTER 6

Getting Unstuck

When you are stuck in a cycle of bad sleep, it's overwhelming. It's so hard to figure out what and how to change to get yourselves on track. You are in pure survival mode: You're trying to get as much sleep as possible, and you're afraid that if you change things, they'll get worse. Or you can't agree on a strategy, so you're doing nothing. You might be blaming each other for the problem, and your anger, fatigue, and resentment are preventing active planning. You dread what it will take to improve things. Or maybe you actually think this is normal. Parenting is all about sleep deprivation, right? Wrong.

You have to do something; it's just not going to get better on its own. You might be coping, but your short-

> Research studies have repeatedly shown that most sleep problems do not resolve on their own. This is not a phase. Do something!

term solutions aren't improving things. They aren't *teaching* your baby how to sleep independently. They aren't getting your baby rested enough for her body to relax into a normal sleep schedule.

It's hard to think clearly and be optimistic when you're so tired and frustrated. And it's hard to stick with a strategy that needs time and persistence when you aren't sure if it's working. The key is to *rely on your new knowledge* of your baby's sleep needs, the biorhythm, the awful effect of overfatigue, and the ways in which you inadvertently reward your baby's waking or protests. Take a step back and assess each of these points. Figure out what's keeping your baby from sleeping and then figure out your plan of attack.

It can't be said often enough: *sleep is a 24-hour process.* Bad naps lead to bad nights and early mornings, which then lead to bad naps. Figuring out where your baby's sleep is getting derailed in the course of the day or night is the first step.

Your Self-Assessment

Use a sleep diary to track your baby's sleep for a week or two. This will help you to identify where things are going wrong. (There is a sample sleep diary in the back of this book.) Healthy babies who aren't sleeping are usually stuck in a combination of some or all of the following problems:

EARLY WAKING. Early waking is any time before 6 a.m. When babies start the day too early, the whole schedule gets off track. They can't stay up long enough to time their naps in sync with the body's natural rhythm. The naps tend to be shorter and less restorative, and extra naps are necessary to fill in the gaps.

YOUR BABY DOESN'T OR WON'T NAP IN THE COT. Overtired babies have a harder time falling and staying asleep. This is especially difficult at nap time. And napping in motion or on another person can interfere with the quality of the nap, leaving the baby prone to overfatigue even when the nap itself seems to be long enough. A 2-hour nap in the stroller can be less restful than a 1-hour nap in the cot. Teaching your baby to nap in the cot is critical for daytime and nighttime sleep.

YOU ARE PUTTING YOUR BABY INTO THE COT ALREADY ASLEEP AT NAP TIME. Babies who are transferred to the cot asleep often have short naps. When they cycle through deep sleep and back into lighter sleep, they become aware of not being held, and they wake up. This leads to short naps and overfatigue. A baby who falls asleep in the cot will learn how to return to deep sleep after completing a full sleep cycle.

YOUR BABY IS TAKING TOO MANY OR TOO FEW NAPS FOR HIS AGE. After 4–5 months of age, babies are programmed to take a certain number of naps. A 5-month-old baby who gets 3–4 hours of daytime sleep in three naps will be better rested than if he got the same amount of sleep in five naps. Having too few naps is a result of imposing a schedule that the baby is not ready for or of simply not understanding the baby's need for sleep.

THE BEDTIME IS TOO LATE. A bedtime that is too late ruins the whole night, causing fussiness and protest during the routine, multiple night wakings, and early mornings. Parents often miss the bedtime cues because overtired babies seem wide awake.

THE BABY DOES NOT FALL ASLEEP IN THE COT AT BEDTIME. Transferring a sleeping baby to the cot gets harder as they get bigger. You can't be as graceful as you were in the beginning. Your baby is more aware of your presence and your desire to put him down. And babies who don't fall asleep in the cot at bedtime have a harder time sleeping through the night. During normal nighttime arousals, they don't know how to fall back to sleep without you.

YOU ARE REINFORCING NIGHT WAKING. Every time you respond to your baby during the night, you are encouraging your baby to wake fully during normal shifts in sleep phases instead of cycling back into deeper sleep independently. Whether you are responding minimally with a dummy replacement or fully by picking her up, rocking, and/or feeding, the effect is the same: you are teaching your child to wake up during the night to get your attention.

AT SOME POINT DURING THE NIGHT, THE BABY ENDS UP IN YOUR BED. Babies often start out in the cot at bedtime only to be brought into their parents' bed at some point. Some parents bring the baby into bed when they go to bed for the night. Others get through multiple wakings before giving up and bringing the baby to bed at 2 or 4 or maybe 5 a.m. Aside from the well-known safety risks of cosleeping, this teaches your baby to wake up more during the night. The trouble here is that the bed becomes the jackpot for the baby. He doesn't necessarily know when he will break you, so he keeps waking until he ends up in your bed. In other words, bringing your baby into your bed on a given night encourages your baby to wake up *more frequently* the next night until you give in again. Even if you hold out until early morning, keep in mind that your baby expects this response from you when he wakes up in the morning. If his wakeup time creeps earlier or night waking increases, the early-morning snuggle is probably the culprit.

YOU ARE DREAM FEEDING. Dream feeding can cause night waking. If you are dream feeding your baby and find that she now wakes up in time for the feeding and/or wakes up at other times during the night, it's time to stop. Remember that once babies are big enough to consume all of their daily calories in a 12-hour span, they will sleep better if you stop feeding at night. Night feeding keeps the digestive system and metabolism active. Allowing the metabolism to naturally slow down at night will make night feeding unnecessary and improve sleep quality.

YOU ARE TREATING THE 4 A.M. WAKING AS MORNING. Unless you live on a farm or deliver newspapers, **4 a.m.**

is not morning. No baby wants to be awake at that time. If you respond to the 4 a.m. waking and start the day, your baby will not learn to go back to sleep.

Determining Your Plan of Action

Now that you have identified your problem areas, you can start planning your intervention. The first question to ask is whether you want to work gradually or aggressively. This seems like a no-brainer: who wants to put a baby through an aggressive sleep-training process if they don't have to?

Well, it's not so simple. Gradual strategies take time and persistence, and they don't necessarily get the results you want or need. Exhausted, desperate parents often find it difficult to stick with a gradual sleep-training plan, especially when a gradual plan sometimes leads to things getting worse before they get better.

Stella: Burned-Out Parents Weighing the Options

Stella, a 9-month-old girl, had not learned to fall asleep in the cot. Her parents transferred her to her cot asleep, which had become a drawn-out and back-breaking process. Stella was waking up at least every 2 hours during the night. Each time, her mother breastfed her back to sleep and moved her into the cot. But at some point during the night, Stella's mother would be too exhausted to get up and would bring her into bed instead of returning her to the cot. At that point, she would feed off and on for the rest of the night.

Stella's parents were exhausted, and the strain was showing in their marriage. They did not want to let Stella cry, but they were at a breaking point. The gradual option would mean less sleep in the short term. First, Stella would be put back into the cot every time she woke up during the night to phase out the expectation of cosleeping. Then, Stella would be soothed back to sleep with less feeding or no feeding, a process that would require teamwork and commitment to long periods of sleeplessness during the night. Then, Stella would be placed in the cot more awake and soothed the rest of the way to sleep without being held.

Going into this process, there was no way to predict how much Stella would protest the changes or how long it would take. There was also the possibility that Stella would become extremely upset when put into the cot awake and that no amount of soothing would get her to sleep without picking her up.

Stella's parents had to determine whether they could invest more sleepless nights indefinitely or tolerate more intense crying in the short term for faster results.

One of the deciding factors in how to proceed is often the number of things that need to change. If a baby is breastfed to sleep, swaddled, dummy-dependent, and cosleeping—that's a lot of changes to make. My bet is that the amount of crying and sleep deprivation using a gradual method in such a case would far exceed what would happen with a cry-it-out approach.

Also consider that you are probably at your worst right now. You might normally be disciplined, resolute, and calm under pressure. But you haven't slept in far too long. You're confused and indecisive. If your strategy requires you to be at your best, you're in trouble. It's no failure or cop-out to decide in favor of tackling the situation head-on.

There is a middle-ground approach, which is to work systematically on a few easily adjusted areas and get your baby as rested as possible. You can probably identify some low-hanging fruit to work on before diving in fully. And then, once you have made the first phase of changes, you can reassess whether to continue on the gradual path or move on to cry-it-out to finish up the job.

Once you have made your self-assessment, you will have a good sense of the problems to tackle. Understand that you might be overwhelmed by the sheer number of steps required to work gradually. If you are ready to plunge ahead into a cry-it-out strategy, go ahead. But if you want to lay a bit more groundwork, consider this phase-in plan.

Working in Phases

Phase 1: Laying the Groundwork

MOVE THE BEDTIME EARLIER. The easiest change to make is the bedtime. There are always some impediments, but you can make this happen. Remember, this is an intervention. Your baby might have to go to bed ridiculously early to break out of this cycle. But once she is in a good 24-hour rhythm, the schedule will settle into something more manageable.

- Watch your baby between 6 and 7:30 p.m. to observe her drowsiness signs. She might perk up at some point, but don't be fooled; she's tired.
- Use your sleep diary to determine how long your baby is awake between her last nap and bedtime. Depending on her age, this interval will vary. But if it is substantially longer than any other period of wakefulness during the day *and* your baby's sleep needs improvement, it's too long. For example, if your 8-month-old baby is typically awake for 2–3 hours between naps and 4–5 hours before bedtime, move the bedtime earlier.
- Plan to move the bedtime earlier for several days. If it's hard to do this on weekdays, start on the

weekend. By Monday night, you might see enough improvement to move it slightly later.

> Believe it or not, changes of even 15–30 minutes can make a difference.

Benjamin: Finding a Way to Move the Bedtime Earlier

Susan and Ted contacted me about their 6-month-old son, Benjamin. Susan and Ted both work long hours, and Benjamin's night waking was exhausting them. Most nights, Ben's parents began his bedtime routine at 8:30 with the hope that he would be asleep at 9. However, Ben was increasingly struggling to fall asleep at bedtime. Many nights, he would not fall asleep until 9:30 or even 10 and he would wake up every few hours. Ben was waking up for the day at 5 a.m., so some nights he was getting just 7 hours of broken sleep—barely enough for an adult and not nearly enough for an infant. Susan and Ted were struggling because they could not bear to miss seeing Ben after work. But Ben's late bedtime wasn't doing anyone any good. The situation was deteriorating, and something had to give.

In our meeting together, I assessed their full 24-hour sleep system. Fortunately, Ben was a good napper, with three solid naps during the day. His last nap, however, ended between 4:30 and 5:00 p.m., leaving a long stretch before bed. Initially, Susan and Ted said it would be impossible to get Ben to bed any earlier. But when we discussed their evenings—racing home to a cranky, exhausted baby and spending the whole evening trying to get him to go to sleep—they started to realize that their needs and Ben's were at odds. As much as they needed to see Ben, the late bedtime and sleep deprivation was crippling the family.

Susan and Ted agreed to give the early bedtime a try. On the weekend, they put Ben to bed between 6:30 and 7 p.m. By Monday, bedtime was smoother, and Ben was waking less frequently during the night. But on Monday, with a return to a late bedtime, they were back where they started. It was clear that 8:30 p.m. was just too late to start the routine. Susan and Ted decided to devote a full week to the early bedtime. They alternated leaving work early to put Ben down by 7 p.m. Over the course of the week, Ben's night waking stopped.

Susan and Ted took a hard look at their work/life balance and decided to make some changes. They agreed to have their trusted caregiver put Ben to bed on Mondays and Thursdays. Susan made arrangements to be home early on Tuesdays and Ted on Wednesdays. They alternated Fridays. Over time, they were able to push the bedtime a little later during the week, to 7:30 p.m., easing some of the rush. On weekends, they continued putting him down closer to 7 p.m. And, now that they are rested and Ben is sleeping until a more reasonable 6:15 a.m., they are able to enjoy mornings with him before work, when Ben is at his cheery best.

This anecdote elicits a lot of different responses. Some people think it's just ridiculous to schedule your life around a baby's sleep. Others find such a work schedule unthinkable. But the vast majority of parents make these kinds of compromises all the time. The specific choices a family makes about careers and child care matter less than the priorities behind those choices. The fact is, when you have a baby, your life balance changes. To keep that balance working for everyone, you all need sleep. And that starts with recognizing what it takes to get your baby the sleep she needs.

The benefit of the early bedtime extends to other problem areas as well. With this single adjustment, you could see improvement in night waking and early waking, and it could start to be easier for your baby to fall asleep in the cot.

MOVE THE NAPS CLOSER TOGETHER. If your baby is not yet 9 months old and takes fewer than three naps, try adding one. Similarly, if your baby is less than 15 months and has dropped to one nap, you could see some improvement by adding a nap. Dropping a nap too soon creates overfatigue all day long. The nap or naps are spread too far apart, allowing the baby to become overtired or wired before sleep. As you now know, that adrenaline can interfere with falling asleep as well as with nap length and quality. So the whole system topples like a house of cards. Naps fall apart and nights follow, or vice versa.

If your baby is a short napper and takes more than the usual number of naps for his age, it is very possible that the naps are too far apart as well. This makes little sense on the surface: if you want your baby to take just three naps, you are probably trying to space them out across the day. But if your baby is overtired, the nap will be short. Starting earlier often lengthens the nap.

Look closely at your baby's schedule. Now that you understand what happens when your baby is awake for too long, does it seem like there's too much time between naps? Try narrowing the time between naps and adding one to fill the gap between the last nap and bedtime.

Keep in mind that this change might be temporary. If your baby is approaching the age of a nap transition, adding a nap might be an interim step to break into the cycle of overfatigue and improve nap quality and nighttime sleep. Once your baby is rested, she might drop that extra nap without a problem.

Stella, Part 2: Naps First

Stella's parents did not feel ready to jump right into a cry-it-out method. Instead, they opted to work on naps first. They started by shortening the interval between naps and trying to transfer

Stella into the cot after she fell asleep in their arms. The short-ened interval was helping to lengthen naps, but Stella was often startled awake by the transfer. After a couple of days of attempts, Stella's parents decided to stop transferring her and to work first on getting her rested. The transfer would come later (as an interim step), or they would use crying to teach her to fall asleep in the cot.

DO THE FIRST NAP OF THE DAY IN THE COT. If your baby does not nap well in the cot, you have to teach him. The first nap of the day is the easiest one to work with. Your baby is at his most rested after waking up for the day. As the day rolls on, he has more and more opportunity to become overtired, making the nap more precarious. Remember: The shortest period of wakefulness is often the time between waking for the day and the first nap. This is counterintuitive but true. While you are teaching your baby to take the first nap of the day in the cot, watch closely for drowsiness cues as early as 1 hour after he wakes for the day.

When you are making these changes, keep the ideal nap schedule in mind, but don't worry if things don't line up perfectly. The first priority is sleeping in the cot. Once he learns to do that, you can shape the schedule to better match his body's natural clock.

KEEP YOUR BABY IN THE COT ALL NIGHT. If you are cosleeping at any point in the night and you want your baby to learn to return to sleep independently, stop bringing her into your bed. This is a tough one for exhausted parents because it means potentially less sleep for you as your baby protests this change. However, your baby must learn that waking will not be rewarded with cosleeping. To do that, she must learn to expect to be in her cot all night no matter what kind of fuss she raises.

The fastest and most effective way to do this is to use a cry-it-out strategy. But if you aren't ready to do that, you can simply commit to doing whatever it takes to get your baby to stay in the cot all night. When you make this change, your baby will wake up more frequently at first. She is used to being brought into your bed when she wakes during the night, so she will keep waking up to try to make that happen. Your job is to soothe her back to sleep without bringing her into your bed. You might start by nursing or feeding and soothing her to sleep in your arms before returning her to the cot. Then gradually start phasing out the feeding and put her into the cot more awake.

Stella, Part 3: No More Cosleeping

After a few days of longer naps, Stella was much happier during the day. The next logical step was to get her sleeping in the cot all night. Again, Stella's parents were not ready to use a full cry-it-out strategy. However, they started to wait and let Stella fuss a bit before responding to her waking. Within a few nights, Stella's sleep had consolidated, and she was down to two night feedings. She also began falling asleep in the cot when put down drowsy at the end of the bedtime routine. Her parents were stunned that she could fall asleep on her own, and this encouraged them to intervene less throughout the night. There were setbacks, however, and some nights Stella protested more than others.

This was not the full solution, but it accomplished a few things. First, Stella learned that she would not be brought into her parents' bed. Second, Stella learned how to fall asleep in the cot even though she was not yet consistently returning to sleep during the night. Third, by letting her fuss and cry a bit, Stella's parents essentially inoculated themselves, making it easier to tolerate some distress (theirs and hers) in service of teaching Stella to sleep.

STOP DREAM FEEDING. This one is simple: just cut it out and see what happens. You can gradually cut millilitres from the feeding (or shorten the amount of feeding time if you are breastfeeding). Or you can just stop altogether. If your baby wakes up later on, you can soothe him back to sleep or let him cry.

Phase 2: It's Time for Crying

You have probably shed more than a tear or two from exhaustion and frustration during this process. No doubt your baby has as well. The fixes I have detailed should improve things, and sometimes they're all that's needed. But often, the final hurdle can be elusive without crying.

How do you gradually teach your baby to fall asleep in the cot when he cries inconsolably despite all of the shushing and patting you can muster? In my opinion, you probably can't teach him gradually. But, more important, there's really no benefit to continuing to try. Your baby is crying a lot. Your baby is not sleeping when he should. Your baby is unable to self-soothe. These things are not changing despite your efforts to twist into a pretzel and give it your all. Your baby is telling you that it's time to let him learn how to sleep by himself.

Your prep work will help you. It was not in vain, or I wouldn't have suggested it. Getting your child as rested as possible and easing her out of some unproductive habits will speed the process.

Letting your baby cry will resolve the trickier parts previously described. Your baby will learn how to fall asleep in the cot. You will stop reinforcing night waking and stop nighttime feedings. Your baby will wake up partially or even fully at normal intervals and put himself back to sleep. You will break the cosleeping habit. And your baby will stay in the cot until at least 6 a.m., ultimately learning to return to sleep after the 4 a.m. trouble spot.

Nights, Naps, or Both?

I've already discussed how cry-it-out works, but the question now is when and how to implement it. In most situations, I recommend starting the cry-it-out process with nighttime sleep. Cry-it-out strategies tend to work faster for nighttime sleep for a few reasons:

1. Physiological and environmental sleep cues are stronger at night, when the baby's body releases melatonin, signaling the body that it is time for an extended stretch of sleep. Darkness is a strong environmental and physiological sleep cue. And the activity level in the household is minimal, providing few opportunities for disruption or stimulation.
2. Nighttime cry-it-out does not have a time limit. Eventually, your baby will sleep. But daytime cry-it-out does have limits. Those limits can stretch out the process, because the baby can end up crying through a whole nap. When you end the nap attempt, you are essentially rewarding the crying.

It takes more repetition for your baby to learn to sleep independently during the day.

3. Teamwork helps. If you and/or your partner are out all day, it can be harder to stay consistent with the nap training. At night, you can go through this together, staying strong for each other when one of you has doubts.

4. Improving nighttime sleep gets the daytime naps off to a better start, because your baby will be well rested. Often, once nights are in better shape, naps improve by virtue of the baby's ability to self-soothe and fall asleep in the cot and because your baby is not exhausted and wired.

Even with these advantages, there are times when it makes sense to start with naps. For example:

- If you can't bear to let your baby cry without a limit, starting with naps can be more manageable. You can use naps to teach your baby to fall asleep in the cot. The process will also help lengthen and consolidate naps over time so that your baby will be better rested overall, paying forward to nighttime sleep.
- If you share a room with your baby, starting with naps can get the ball rolling while you set up a temporary fix for nighttime sleep training.

- If your baby still needs multiple feedings during the night or you're not ready to night-wean her, working on naps can improve things while you prepare for nights.

How to Use Crying at Nap Time

There are several options for cry-it-out with naps. Whichever option you choose, start with the first nap of the day.

Option 1: Go Whole Hog

This option is the purest and the one most likely to get the quickest results.

- After your nap routine, put your baby down in the cot awake and leave.
- Let her cry for 1 hour.
- If she doesn't sleep, get her up and keep her awake for 1 hour.
- If your baby takes a short nap (less than 40 minutes), let her cry for 15–20 more minutes to give her the opportunity to go back to sleep.

Consistency gets faster results when using cry-it-out at nap time. Remember: Babies can't decipher your rules. You might have a great rationale for letting your baby cry at certain times but not others, but your baby just knows that *sometimes* crying gets her what she wants (you), and that just encourages her to cry *every* time. If crying at nap times *never* gets the desired result, she'll stop trying.

- Put your baby down for the next nap when you see drowsiness cues (after a minimum of 1 hour awake).
- Repeat for every nap.

If your baby has a lot of stamina, this could mean a lot of crying during the day. Typically, if a baby cries through the full nap, she will fall asleep on the second try, but there is often some crying before each nap.

Option 2: Work on the First Nap Only

If you can't face the prospect of multiple nap protests during the day, start with just the first nap. This will take longer, but you have to start somewhere. Often, after a couple of days of working on the first nap, parents feel more prepared to go all out.

Option 3 (for Three-Nap Babies)

Work on all naps at home until 3 p.m., then take a walk for a final stroller nap. The rationale here is to catch up a bit at the end of the day, so that your baby isn't woefully overtired at bedtime. By doing the catch-up nap in a different environment, your baby still has the consistency of going into the cot awake for every nap at home.

Option 4: Force the Schedule

An alternative to the "1-hour-down/1-hour-up" strategies above is to force a nap schedule that approximates the appropriate schedule for your baby's age. I typically prefer to start by allowing more naps at shorter intervals because forcing the schedule can lead to even more over-fatigue. If your baby cries through a nap from 9 to 10 a.m., she would have to wait 2 more hours before the next attempt. That's a long time, and your baby is more likely to fall asleep unintentionally before the next nap time.

However, sticking to the schedule will limit the amount of crying you have to face. Some parents find it easier to approach cry-it-out for naps with a fixed number of nap attempts. Also, when naps are too short and frequent, forcing the schedule can help to consolidate them. I always start by trying to limit overfatigue to allow naps to lengthen naturally. But when that doesn't get the desired results, forcing the schedule can get the job done.

The three-nap schedule for nap training is 9 a.m., 12 p.m., and 3 p.m.

The two-nap schedule is 10 a.m. and 2 p.m.

Remember: While nap training, be prepared for an early bedtime. Days can be rough, and the early bedtime will help your baby recuperate at night.

Stella, Part 4: Cry-It-Out

After she had made significant progress in lengthening her naps, having learned to sleep in her cot all night with less night waking and night feeding, Stella hit a plateau. She was not able to nap well in the cot, and she continued to be unpredictable at night. Some nights, she would put herself back to sleep, and sometimes she would be easily soothed. But there were nights when she was awake and protesting for the better part of several hours. Ultimately, her parents decided that they were ready to take the final leap.

Stella's parents decided to let her cry it out at night first. On the first night, her parents put her down at 6:30 p.m. She cried for 45 minutes and then fell asleep. At midnight, she cried for 90 minutes. She woke briefly around 4:30 a.m. without significant crying and went back to sleep until 7:30. The second night, she went to sleep without crying at bedtime, cried out briefly in the early part of the night, and slept through the night for a total of 12 hours. On subsequent nights, there were occasional short bursts of crying, but that, too, improved quickly.

What If Crying Doesn't Work?

While the vast majority of babies respond to extinction methods of sleep training combined with a focus on preventing overfatigue, there are rare cases in which babies don't respond fully or at all. Working with babies is especially challenging because—of course—they cannot communicate verbally. And I often work with babies before other challenges, such as sensory issues, developmental delays, neurocognitive issues like attention deficit disorder, food sensitivities and allergies, and autism—all of which can affect sleep—become apparent.

This is not to say that all babies who seem resistant to sleep training have huge challenges ahead. Most people who contact me believe that their children are bad sleepers who won't respond to behavioral interventions, and most of them are wrong. There are some babies who are more challenging than others, and it is harder for their parents to stick to a plan when they aren't getting the rapid results that other parents have claimed.

Nora: The Third Time's the Charm

Nora was 5 months old when her exhausted parents contacted me. Her sleep was predictable only in that it was bad. Naps were often as short as 20 minutes, and she was often awake for most of the day. Nights were brutal, with frequent and extended (hours-long) night waking. She was clearly exhausted, but she just wouldn't sleep. Her parents had attempted cry-it-out twice but stopped because Nora was capable of crying for hours and seemed clingy the next day.

When we met, Nora's parents were skeptical about whether I could help. But they were desperate and willing to try anything. Because cry-it-out seemed impossible to the parents, we began by working on Nora's naps.

First, we tried putting her down for naps every 90 minutes. This was grueling work because Nora fought every time and often outlasted her parents' efforts. After a few difficult days, we switched to forcing the nap schedule, working on the assumption that Nora would sleep better if naps were timed to her natural biorhythm. This failed as well.

At night, Nora's waking persisted, and her parents grew more exhausted and hopeless. With the failure of the nap intervention, we would have to work on nights. Gradual strategies had not worked; Nora became agitated if her parents were present but not holding her. Leaving her to fuss and returning to console her agitated her as well. And leaving her to cry to sleep had not been successful because Nora outlasted her parents' resolve.

Finally, it was clear from all of these failures that Nora was not going to learn to sleep with any strategy that felt reasonable. But continuing with her level of sleep deprivation was not feasible either. We decided to let her cry it out again, this time with the expectation that she would fully test her parents' resolve. And she did.

The first night went like this:

6:30 p.m. bedtime
6:30–8 p.m. cry
8–8:30 p.m. sleep
8:30–9 p.m. cry
9–11:45 p.m. sleep
11:45 p.m.–4 a.m. cry
4–6 a.m. cry, with increasing periods of quiet
6:10 a.m. sleep
8:20 a.m. wake

Any reasonable person would give up in this situation. It seems cruel and outrageous to let a child cry that long. However, this was a last-ditch effort for a child who seemed unable to get the sleep she needed. Her parents had steeled themselves for a very tough road because they weren't ready to settle for chronic sleep deprivation.

On night two, Nora cried for 45 minutes and slept for almost 12 hours. On night three, she cried for 15 minutes and slept for 11 hours. Naps took longer to resolve, but Nora's parents persisted, and she settled into a healthy sleep schedule after about a month.

Nora's parents could have easily given up, and I wouldn't have blamed them. But by eliminating all of the alternatives, they became convinced that it was worth one final and heroic shot at teaching Nora to sleep. It was a true act of bravery on their part, and it changed the course of their experience as new parents. They were able to find solid footing and finally enjoy their new family.

In my experience, even in the most challenging cases, cry-it-out works at least partially. If parents truly give it a chance to work by not responding to crying for 2 to 3 nights, babies do learn to fall asleep. Some babies continue to cry for 10 to 30 minutes at bedtime and for short bursts during the night. But when evaluating whether sleep training "works," we must always consider the starting point. Yes, we all want a baby who goes to bed happily, coos himself to sleep, and is silent until a very hospitable morning hour. Some babies do that. Others fuss and cry but get the sleep they need, and it's far more and better sleep than they were getting before they learned to fall asleep alone.

Where things get trickier is around 4 a.m. Most babies have trouble around 4 a.m. at one point or another. It is often the last burst of night waking/crying to fade away. Overtired babies often wake up at 4 a.m. and have trouble going back to sleep. And some babies just seem to be unable to go back to sleep at all once 4 a.m. rolls around. In very difficult cases, it can take weeks of sleep training to work this out. And in some cases, it seems that nothing works.

Before you throw in the towel and declare your child a bad sleeper, make sure that you have really devoted yourself to sleep training. Have you been utterly consistent? Is your child going to bed overtired, which easily undermines nighttime sleep? Are you reinforcing the protests or night waking some—or all—of the time? If there is really nothing left to try, it's time to consider whether something else is causing the problem.

First, talk to your doctor about known physiological causes of sleep problems. Simple things like low iron levels can cause sleep problems. Chronic ear infections, sleep apnea, and enlarged tonsils or adenoids are also frequent culprits.

Take a holistic view as well. Are you adhering to a special diet while breastfeeding? Are you taking medication? Are you raising your child vegan? These things have different effects on different children. Also consider sleep problems in the context of other issues like eczema, reflux, or early sensory sensitivities like extreme distress over clothing changes, baths, or temperature fluctuations. You might need to treat or correct the underlying cause to see improvement in sleep.

If you are stuck, think outside the box. Acupuncture, osteopathy, chiropractic, or craniosacral treatments may be helpful. These are options to research in your community and discuss with your doctor. The scientific literature is lacking when it comes to a lot of alternative health-care practices, but there are many highly skilled practitioners out there who can help you to identify otherwise overlooked sources of the problem.

Key Points from Chapter 6

- The vast majority of sleep problems result from overfatigue, inability to self-soothe, and habits reinforced by parents' attempts to help.
- An early bedtime and restorative naps are essential for nighttime sleep.
- Once you identify the source of the problem, you can determine whether it makes sense to take gradual steps or to move straight to cry-it-out.
- Letting your baby cry teaches her to fall asleep independently, so that she will be able to return to sleep independently during normal nighttime arousals.

CHAPTER 7

Tricky Circumstances

While everything might make sense to you now, you still might have trouble figuring out how to make all of these strategies work in your life. Your situation has specific elements and constraints that have to be incorporated or accommodated. At first glance, it might seem impossible.

One of the benefits of doing home visits is that I really get to understand the particular challenges that each family is dealing with. I don't go as far as carrying my own tape measure, but I have helped parents fit cots into spots they never imagined would work. When you are sleep deprived, your thinking is much less flexible and creative. It's important to take a step back and consider all possibilities before crossing anything off the list.

> It might seem like raising a good sleeper requires round-the-clock vigilance and homebound commitment to sleep. But the point of all of this is not to make you sleep obsessed. Instead, the information here will enable you to create a framework for good sleep, eliminating unintentional missteps and incorporating some key changes that make a big difference. Balance, flexibility, and creativity are important.

In my work as a sleep consultant, I tailor treatment plans to meet the needs of each family's circumstances, outlining priorities and finding wiggle room where no one thought it possible. Although no book can provide alternatives for every contingency, I will address some common challenges that face many families. You can find a way to get unstuck even when competing demands and constraints feel as if they can never be reconciled.

Space Challenges

I live and work in New York City, where some families have spacious apartments or townhouses with rooms to spare but where many others are making it work in studios or one-bedroom apartments. In a perfect world, a baby would have her own room or one to share with a sibling, but that's not always possible.

The first step is to figure out whether you need a short-term or long-term solution. If you are planning to move in the near future, your temporary solution does not have to be pretty. Your baby can sleep in a closet, extra bathroom, or even a corner cordoned off by a screen or curtain. Or maybe you can tough it out on a sofa bed or air mattress in the living room while your baby sleeps in the bedroom.

Even if you need a more permanent solution, go with a temporary one first to get your baby well rested and, ideally, sleeping through the night. Once your baby is sleeping well, you will have a better idea of what he needs to *keep* sleeping well. You might very well be able to share a room with your baby once he is in a good rhythm. But if you find that your baby is too sensitive to your presence even when he otherwise can sleep through the night, it's time to find something more permanent. Think about ways to put a barrier between your bed and the cot. Consider a temporary wall or half-wall to divide the space. Use white noise to create a sound barrier. Get blackout shades to make it very dark. If you find yourself stuck, ask a friend to look at your situation with fresh eyes or consult with a designer.

Siblings

When you have the needs of two or more kids to balance, you'll be making some compromises. Do not judge yourself or feel guilty about depriving one or another of your children of perfect parenting. There are certainly benefits to getting a parent's undivided attention, but there are also tremendous benefits to having a sibling. Using *The Good Sleeper* principles gives you the foundation for choosing your compromises wisely.

And it's usually not as grim as you think. Parents with older children often feel guilty when they realize how much less attention they can devote to a new baby. Compared to the attention the firstborn received, it seems like younger siblings will surely grow up with some kind of neglect complex. But such fears are overblown. And as challenging as it can be to protect an infant's sleep when you have older children, there are some sleep-related advantages for younger siblings.

For example, you will have to put your younger baby down much more than you did her older sibling. As a result, she will get used to sleeping somewhere other than in your arms much sooner than your older child might have. You will also have to let your baby fuss and cry sometimes. There will be times when your baby is unhappy about being put down and you won't be able to do anything but leave her for a few minutes to keep your toddler from tearing up the place. Sometimes, by the time you get back to her, your baby will be calm or asleep.

However, she will also be doing a lot of sleeping on the go. When you are at home, she can sleep in the cot or moses basket. But you will also be entertaining an older child who needs to get out of the house. This is not much of an issue during the early weeks because your newborn can sleep anywhere. But as she becomes more stimulated by her surroundings, her sleep quality will be affected. Here are a few strategies to help you juggle:

1. Try to stay home until after your baby's first nap of the day. This essentially assures that your baby will get one solid nap.
2. Use the stroller instead of a carrier for at least some naps on the go. **Napping in the carrier is harder to phase out because the baby grows dependent on physical contact.**
3. Whenever possible, park the stroller while your baby is sleeping. Minimizing movement improves sleep quality.
4. Compensate with an early bedtime so that nighttime sleep is not affected.

As your younger child settles into a nap schedule and is old enough to sleep through the night, you will get a better sense of her particular needs and where you can push her to be more flexible. You might find that one nap is more important than the others or that by a certain time of day, your baby is overstimulated and can't nap outside. You also might have specific constraints that require you to be out at certain times, such as needing to drop your older child at school or pick that child up. In those cases, you have to figure out how best to compensate.

Bedtime is another challenge when you have more than one child. Parents often struggle with the evening schedule, trying to manage an older child who probably can't be left unattended and who needs to eat, bathe, and be entertained while attending to a baby who needs to go to bed early.

The key is getting your baby down for the night first, so that you can focus your attention on the older child. Your older child can participate in the routine to a point, but you will probably need to have some way for her to be safely occupied elsewhere for 10–15 minutes while you finish your baby's bedtime routine. That's not hard if your older child can be left alone. But if you have a toddler, you'll need a play yard, a very safe room, or another person to help you. Neighborhood teenagers and even tweens can be a great help in these times. You just need someone to pop in and keep your child occupied and safe for a short amount of time.

Room Sharing

I am a firm believer in room sharing among siblings. Kids generally enjoy sharing a room, and it can be good for them. Not only do they get to have a companion, but they also learn to respect each other's needs (i.e., sleep). Sharing a room helps them to develop their own relationship by spending time together without parents around. One day, you'll wake up to hear your kids chatting in the morning instead of calling for you. That's the positive side.

But room sharing presents a challenge for sleep training. For the most part, your kids won't disturb each other during the night even if there's a fair amount of crying. However, crying at bedtime or in the early morning can be disruptive. And you are likely to be very anxious about your baby waking your older child, making it harder for you to leave your baby to fuss and cry to sleep.

SLEEP TRAINING IN A SHARED ROOM. When you are teaching your baby to sleep through the night, it's easier if you aren't also worrying about disrupting your older child. If you are using a cry-it-out method to teach your baby to sleep through the night, the easiest method is to move your older child out of his bedroom temporarily while you sleep-train your baby in the kids' room. Your older child could sleep on a mattress on the floor of your room, for example. If he is still using a cot himself, you could set up a portable cot somewhere else or even move his cot if it has wheels. Explain that he will be camping out while the baby learns to sleep.

Kids usually love this. But if you think your older child will love this idea too much and it will be hard to get him back into his room when the time comes, have him camp out in the living room. Or put your baby in your room to sleep-train, sleep in the living room yourselves, and keep your older child in his room for the process. Even better, if you have the opportunity, send your older child to stay with Grandma or have one parent take him away for a weekend while the other supervises the sleep training at home.

Explain to your older child that the baby will cry sometimes in her sleep. If your older child is very sensitive, you can give him the option of going to your room and sleeping on your floor when the baby wakes him (provided this won't create a new set of problems).

Putting your baby to bed first helps. That way, you can let her fuss if necessary without disturbing your older child. You can do your older child's routine in another room. If all goes well, your baby will be fast asleep by the time your older child goes to bed.

TACKLING EARLY WAKING IN A SHARED ROOM. Your later sleeper will be more vulnerable to his sibling's crying as it gets closer to morning, so it's harder to ignore early waking. However, responding to early waking reinforces it, making it more likely to become a pattern. First, try

an earlier bedtime for a few days to see if the early waking is caused by overfatigue. If that doesn't solve the
problem, you can let your baby cry in the morning.
Things might get harder before they get better if your
older child is disturbed by the noise. Decide whether it
makes more sense to move your older child out of the
room preemptively for several days or to just deal with
the disruption when it happens. Your days with your older
child will start earlier than you want while you get your
baby on track. But persistence will get you unstuck.

NAPPING IN A SHARED ROOM. This can be tricky if you are
putting both kids down at the same time. If you find that
they keep each other up, put your baby in a portable cot
in another room for naps or let your older child sleep on
your bed.

Dean: Ending the 4 a.m. Dummy Game
(and Preserving an Older Sibling's Sleep)

*Dean had made it through colic and was sleeping through the
night by 4 months of age without much in the way of crying.
But when he was about 6 months old, he started waking more
fully at 4 a.m. Initially, his parents were able to go in, replace his
dummy, and he'd go back to sleep until 6:30. This was unpleas-
ant but manageable in the short term because Dean's parents
were trying to keep him from waking his older sister.*

But over the course of a couple of weeks, Dean stopped going back to sleep so easily. He'd quiet down for 10–15 minutes, but then he'd spit out the dummy and cry some more. Eventually, Dean and his parents were essentially awake from 4 to 6 a.m., with tiny increments of dozing between dummy placements. This was awful for Dean and unsustainable for Dean's parents, who both had demanding jobs.

Fortunately, a three-day weekend was coming up. Dean's dad took his sister away for the weekend while his mother stayed home to attack the sleep problem. On the first night, Dean cried for 40 minutes at 4 a.m. and went back to sleep. He cried for 20 minutes on the second and third nights. With his sister back in her own bed on the fourth night, Dean's parents almost threw in the towel. But they stuck it out. Dean cried—really screamed— for 15 minutes. His sister slept through it. And on the fifth night, there was no crying at all.

Travel

Good sleepers want to sleep, and that works to everyone's advantage when traveling. In an ideal world, you can take some sleep cues with you such as white noise (phone apps work well for travel) or music. And in that ideal world, it's easier to stick to the schedule.

But the reality of travel is that it is challenging when you're with a child. You have to bring *so much stuff*. And while you want to have a good time, you don't get a vacation from being a parent. Here are some tips to make the best of it:

- Bring a familiar-smelling item for the cot, like the unwashed cot sheet.
- Bring white noise. This is a potent sleep cue for your baby, and it will help her sleep in a new place. It will also give you some peace of mind when doors slam, glasses clink, or people start having a noisy good time.
- Do not cosleep. Make sure that your baby has a safe and separate place to sleep. Hotels often have cots, although they vary in quality. There are also resources in many places for renting baby gear. If you are visiting friends or family, ask them if they have contacts who might be willing to lend a travel cot or if they can tap into a local parenting network on your behalf.
- Even if you have to sleep in the room with your baby, make sure there's a somewhat separate space to hang out while the baby is sleeping. Otherwise, you'll be sitting in the dark or watching movies on your laptop in the bathroom after your baby goes to sleep.
- Stick to the schedule as much as possible, but don't let it rule you; have fun, too.

- Make sure your baby gets at least some good naps. Consider it an investment in everyone's enjoyment of the trip.
- Get a babysitter. You won't have fun with a screaming baby at a fancy restaurant, so plan ahead.
- Don't push your baby too much at once. If you've had a hard day of travel, make sure to get your baby to bed at a reasonable time. Don't skip multiple naps in a row. If you have a hard-charging day, plan a more restful one the following day.
- Get help! Talk to your travel companions in advance about what you need. Trade off primary baby duties so you can enjoy yourself, too. Explore babysitting options in advance.
- Your baby might need more soothing at bedtime, but don't overdo it. Don't assume that your baby will be frightened or disoriented. Ask yourself whether your help is helping. If not, back off and let your baby fuss or cry to settle down.
- If your baby wakes up in the night, you can check on her if you think it would be helpful, but don't spend lots of time trying to soothe her. You will probably just be agitating her. It's okay to let her cry—location permitting—away from home.
- Don't resume night feeding if you have already stopped. If you must soothe your baby (and that

is a big *if*), try everything possible to avoid feeding.

- Get back on track as soon as possible when you get home. Don't get caught feeling guilty about having disrupted things with your vacation. Just get your baby back on schedule. Let her cry if necessary. Remember: The sooner you let her cry to get back on track, the faster you will see results. If you wait, you are just establishing new and counterproductive expectations that you'll have to quash.
- Whenever possible, plan to have an extra day of vacation at home before returning to work. The buffer day will give you time to readjust to your normal routine and your baby's before you add the stress of work.

The harsh reality of travel with a child is that it's not as relaxing as it was before you had her. You can't just kick back and get a complete break from all of your responsibilities. It's important to manage your expectations and think ahead about the kind of vacation you want to have. Do you want the privacy of a house on the beach where you do the cooking and cleaning, or do you want to find an all-inclusive option? What do you need a break from in your daily life? If you are clear about your needs and desires, you will make better choices.

That said, travel is important. **If you live in fear of disrupting your baby's rhythm, you will miss out on too much.** Your baby will benefit from time spent away from home, from meeting relatives, and from having some quality time with you. Disruptions can be worth it. And you now know what you need to do to get back on track if things need fixing when you get home.

Jet Lag

Travel is one thing, but jet lag throws in a bit of a wrench. If you are traveling across one or two time zones, your baby probably won't notice. You can adjust the bedtime to split the difference. But if you are traveling across several time zones, the transition can be trickier.

You can't force your baby to sleep, but you can keep him awake to set his body clock to local time. Wake him up in the morning close to the usual time. And make sure to wake him from naps so he doesn't sleep too long. Use your baby's typical nap schedule as a guide. If a nap is usually 2 hours at home, wake him after a 2-hour nap on vacation to help his body adjust to the new time. The danger is that he will take a nap and continue sleeping as though it is nighttime, only to be wide awake in the middle of the night. **Note: This is a specific strategy for dealing with jet lag. It does not apply to normal napping at home.**

When your baby is awake during the day, get outside. Natural light and fresh air help the body adjust to local time, in part by suppressing the release of melatonin that signals bedtime. Plan to be active when your baby should be awake and do your best to prevent unintentional naps.

Chances are, there will be some night waking at odd times. Do your best not to reinforce this with feeding. If your baby is really up for the day in the middle of the night, *someone* will have to occupy her. Plan ahead and take turns with the nighttime burden so no one ends up feeling cheated out of a vacation.

Daylight Savings

Similar to jet lag, daylight savings can be a bit tricky. On the surface, the 1-hour time change seems negligible. In fact, most babies will adjust to the new time within a week. But that week can be exhausting for parents, and it's important to keep your child from becoming overtired. Here are some strategies to avoid common pitfalls.

PREPARE BY SPLITTING THE DIFFERENCE. For a couple of days before and after the time change, alter your child's schedule by 30 minutes to make the shift more gradual. In the spring, prepare by putting your baby to bed 30 minutes earlier for nights and naps. When the clocks "spring forward," put your baby to bed 30 minutes *after* the usual time for a few days. Then go back to the usual time. Confused? If your baby's bedtime is 7 p.m., you will put her down at 6:30 p.m. before DST and 7:30 p.m. after DST to help her adjust. Then you can go back to 7 p.m. In the autumn, do the opposite: put your baby down 30 minutes later before the clocks change and 30 minutes earlier afterward. Then revert to the regular bedtime.

DON'T IGNORE THE CHANGE IN TIME. Parents often try to keep their babies on the "old" time, particularly in the spring, when they hope to gain a later bedtime and morning wake-up. Wouldn't it be nicer if your baby slept from 8 p.m. to 7 a.m. instead of 7 p.m. to 6 a.m.? Yes it would, but it's unlikely to work for long. I am not aware of any scientific studies that explain this phenomenon in children, but I have seen it demonstrated by countless babies who became overtired when their parents stuck with a later bedtime after "springing forward." The body usually adjusts to the local time even if you try to shift everything forward. And keeping your baby awake too late will result in overfatigue.

The one exception is for babies who wake up very

The impact of Daylight Savings Time on infant and toddler circadian rhythms has not been well studied. It seems reasonable to expect—or hope—that the shift forward in springtime would give parents a respite from the early bedtime/earlier-than-pleasant wake time schedule. If the sun stays out later, melatonin release should be delayed, making bedtime naturally later. So why do sleep problems arise when parents try to stick with a later bedtime in summer? My guess is that it's schedule and activity related.

Regardless of wake-up times, nap times tend to stay constant, especially as naps decrease to twice and then once a day. Activity schedules are centered on these nap times and don't tend to shift forward with DST. With the nap ending at the usual time and the bedtime pushed later, the baby is awake for too long before bed. He gets overtired, which often causes early waking, throwing him further off the schedule. Kids are also more active in spring and summer, making them *more* tired in the evening even when they seem full of energy. And parents get sloppier about bedtimes when it's nice out. I do it, too.

You can avoid trouble simply by staying aware of your child's need for sleep. If pushing the schedule later seems to work, that's fine. Just make sure to adjust if you start to notice signs of overfatigue. Don't stick with a later bedtime if you notice that your baby is struggling to settle at bedtime, starts waking during the night, or gets up too early in the morning. And if you make it through the summer with a later bedtime, don't forget to switch back to an earlier bedtime when Daylight Savings ends in the autumn. Your baby will be waking up earlier then, and the early bedtime will prevent overfatigue.

early and have to go to bed very early to compensate. In this case, Daylight Savings Time can work to your advantage to help your baby get on a more normal schedule. If your baby is already overtired by a 6 p.m. bedtime, the shift forward will help. You'll be able to put him to bed at 6 p.m. after the time change, but his body will read it as 5 p.m. and he won't yet be overtired.

TEACH YOUR BABY TO GO TO BED EVEN THOUGH IT'S STILL LIGHT OUTSIDE. Bedtimes creep later in the summer for a variety of reasons. Parents often say that their kids can't go to sleep when it's still light out. And some of us happen to enjoy staying out at a summer barbecue past 6 p.m. Keeping your baby up late occasionally isn't going to wreak havoc beyond the immediate (possible) effect of overfatigue. But consistently letting your child stay up until dark during the summer is going to lead to problems.

It's true that it's easier to go to bed when it's dark. But babies can learn to go to sleep when it's still light out. It's up to the parents to send the right messages. First, if you haven't done so already, get some dark shades or curtains. Your baby's body will respond to the darkness in her room even if the sun is still blazing. Second, don't fall for the delay tactics. Parents tend to lose their resolve in the summer and let things slide. Routines get drawn out and time (and sleep) is lost. Parents forget what they know about adrenaline. Instead, they think the baby isn't tired at bedtime because she doesn't *look* tired. But those bursts of energy at night mean the same thing regardless of the sun—overfatigue. So put your baby to bed!

Changes and Derailments

Once your baby is sleeping, you might find yourself getting anxious about rocking the boat. That's normal, but you're going to have to get over it. Developmental milestones pop up, throwing curves into routines. And life intervenes with all sorts of extraordinary circumstances like illness, stress, schedule changes, child-care adjustments, and the like. It's important to pay attention to these challenges, but don't panic. Good sleepers can recover from disruptions and change.

Illness

It is stressful and often frightening when babies get sick. They can't communicate verbally, and you are left trying to determine whether a fever is just a fever or an indication of something more. It takes time to learn how your baby handles illness. Some babies sleep right through coughing and sniffles, whereas others have a much harder time. As a rule, sleep training takes a backseat to illness. If your baby needs you, help her. Remember: When you are leaving your baby alone to self-soothe it is because she *doesn't* need you. So respond to the need.

Keep in mind, however, that your help might be depriving your baby of sleep she needs to get well. If your help isn't helping, your baby might still be better off fussing or crying herself to sleep. If your baby is mildly ill and you are providing comfort only, it's possible that she will get more sleep if you leave her alone. But if your baby needs your attention—if she has a stomach virus and needs fluids or if she has respiratory problems and needs a nebulizer, for example—you cannot leave her alone. This is a case-by-case situation that should be discussed with your doctor.

Good sleepers often rally naturally after an illness. But if they don't give up the night waking on their own, it is up to you to get them back on track. As with travel or any disruption, return to your routines as soon as possible. Letting your baby cry for a sleep-training tune-up will not be as intense as it was the first time you let her cry *if you do it sooner rather than later.*

Teething

Teething is a little more ambiguous. Many doctors say that teething isn't painful. I'm not so sure about that, having looked into the minefield of my kids' mouths as they cut several molars at a time and recalling the change in their dispositions once the worst of each teething episode had passed. However, teething doesn't have to destroy sleep. Good sleepers tend to be less bothered by less intense teething when it comes to sleep. But those intense, multiple-tooth episodes can cause trouble. Bedtime might be harder, and night waking can reemerge, especially around 4 a.m.

Because teething is less isolated than illness, it's important to limit your nighttime interventions. When you know your child is in pain, you can treat it. Talk to your doctor about options for pain management. But don't get into the habit of long nursing, rocking, or walking sessions to get your baby back to sleep. These interactions become stimulating and encourage more night waking. Teething babies can sleep, and it's not cruel to let them fuss or cry in service of that sleep.

Developmental Milestones

Your baby is constantly growing and acquiring new skills, and these changes can cause temporary setbacks when it comes to sleep. The key word here is *temporary*. As long as you don't panic, his sleep can get back on track quickly.

Rolling, standing, walking, and talking are the major developments that can disrupt sleep. When your baby learns to roll from back to front, he will be surprised and frustrated. He'll fuss, cry, and have trouble falling back to sleep initially. Once he is rolling over, you should immediately stop swaddling. On his belly, your baby needs access to his arms to push up and reposition himself. Go through your SIDS safety checklist and make absolutely sure that the cot is free of all possible suffocation hazards (i.e., firm mattress, no loose bedding, no fluffy bumpers, no stuffed animals, no sleeping on soft sofas or other furniture). Once your baby is rolling to his belly independently, it is considered safe to leave him there. However, it's always a good idea to check with your doctor if you have safety concerns, especially if your baby is younger than 3 months old.

Always put your baby into the cot on his back, even if he is able to roll onto his belly.

The first few times your baby rolls over at night, you will probably go in and put him on his back. This might help initially, and some doctors recommend doing it for a few nights. But as he refines his rolling, he'll begin flipping right back to his belly even if he's not very happy when he gets there. He simply has to get used to sleeping on his belly. Once he does, it will probably become his preferred position.

The best and fastest way to help your baby adjust to sleeping on his stomach is to leave him alone. Yes, he'll cry and fuss, but he will learn to get comfortable. Some parents prefer to try patting and shushing before reverting to letting the baby cry. But remember, whenever you go to your baby to "help," you risk waking the baby fully and setting up his expectation of getting attention during the night. Your baby could quickly turn the waking into a habit instead of returning to independent self-soothing. Leave him alone, and he'll adjust to this new development quickly. It generally takes about a week for babies to fully adjust to their new rolling talents.

Similarly, when your baby learns to stand, she will need to learn to return to sitting and lying down. By the time your baby is standing, she is much more stimulated by you, especially during the night. Going to her to help her sit or lie down can quickly turn into a game, a game that is no fun for you in the middle of the night. Babies who stand in the cot might even fall asleep standing initially, but they will lie down eventually. In most cases, that happens quickly. But even if your baby continues to stand, going in to help is likely to backfire. If you are convinced that your baby does not know how to sit down from a standing position, practice during the day, when it's appropriate to play games.

Walking and talking are also big developments that

can impact sleep. The increases in cognitive and physical activity are very likely to overstimulate the baby and can make it hard for her to settle down. Keep in mind that these developments are *exhausting*, and your baby might need more sleep to help him through these transitions. **Move the bedtime earlier even if your baby doesn't seem tired.** Remember, all that excitement is likely to involve adrenaline, so your baby might be overtired.

Kevin: Standing Up All Night

Kevin was a 22-month-old boy who could not sleep through the night. Because of some serious medical issues in infancy, his parents deferred sleep training. By the time they contacted me, the medical issues had been resolved, but Kevin was unable to fall asleep in the cot or sleep through the night. What were once brief waking episodes had lengthened into long breastfeeding sessions and reluctant cosleeping.

We started by making the usual changes to Kevin's schedule and routines. Things improved, but Kevin continued to wake up during the night. Although his parents returned him to the cot and stopped feeding him during the night, his nighttime protests persisted with intensity. His parents decided to let him cry.

On the first night of letting him cry, Kevin's parents tried doing Ferber-style checking on a schedule. Each time he woke up, he would stand up. His parents alternated going in and lay-

ing him down, but he popped back up immediately. This went on for hours.

The next night, Kevin's parents decided not to check on him. To their surprise, he cried for less than an hour but fell asleep standing up. They went in to lay him down, but he woke up and cried for another 2 hours.

The following night, Kevin cried at bedtime and again fell asleep standing up, this time with his arms over the sides of the cot to keep him upright. His parents realized that intervening at all would prolong the process, so they did not go in. Although they did not watch continuously, it seemed the next day that Kevin had slept standing up all night.

I must confess that I was very worried about this. I had never encountered such fortitude before, and I really had no idea how it would turn out. But in our many discussions throughout the process, Kevin's parents and I kept coming back to the fact that going in to help was not actually helping Kevin. They stuck it out and, after three more days of sleeping upright, Kevin started lying down to sleep and staying there happily all night.

Developmental Changes to the Sleep Schedule

At various points, your baby's sleep schedule and bio-rhythm will change. Sometime between 8 and 10 months of age, your baby will drop the third nap and establish a two-nap schedule. Between the ages of 14 and 18 months, she'll move to a single-nap schedule. And sometime between the ages of 3 and 5 years, she'll stop napping altogether.

Whenever a child begins to get less sleep during the day, she is likely to become overtired before bed. That often results in a new round of bedtime protests, night waking, and/or early waking. This is so common, especially at the 8-month mark, that it has been dubbed the *8-month regression*. But this regression almost invariably coincides with a dropped nap, so it is more apt to call it overfatigue. Remember this always: **Whenever your baby grows out of a nap, make the bedtime earlier.** Getting your baby to bed before she is dramatically overtired will smooth out the adjustment process. Over time, the bedtime will edge later, when your baby is well rested.

Key Points from Chapter 7

- You do not have to live in a perfect world to have a good sleeper. Space constraints, siblings, schedule disruptions, and developmental milestones can all be overcome.
- With any disruption or development, there are two rules of thumb:

- ▶ First, keep your baby well rested by protecting naps and making the bedtime earlier if necessary.
- ▶ Second, avoid reinforcing the disruption with too much help or attention. Your good sleeper might get used to seeing you, and that will encourage the behavior you're trying to leave behind.
- When schedules and routines get derailed (e.g., illness, travel), reset as soon as possible.
- Letting your child cry it out to get back to formerly great habits will work quickly. It is rarely as difficult as it was the first time around.

CHAPTER 8

Child Care

The issue of child care—whether, how much, what sort—is yet another source of anxiety among new parents. There are a lot of opinions these days about how parents, and women in particular, should be engaged in the workplace and at home. And those opinions run the gamut. Some are based solely on tradition or emotion. Others are based on economics. And still others stem from the science of child development.

I'm not going to pretend to be impartial here. I'm a working mother and therefore avail myself of child care. But in the years I've been working with new parents, I have seen it done in just about every way. Even when one parent becomes a full-time caregiver, setting up some form of child care not only gives the parent a break, but it also helps the parent to step back and learn to let other people take care of the baby. My goal is to provide the information you need to make an informed choice instead of an emotional one.

I always planned to return to work after having kids because I knew that my professional identity gave me one sort of fulfillment I needed. But as my first maternity leave wound down just as my son became a lot more fun to be around, I began to feel desperate about handing him over to someone else so soon. The reality of the impending separation broke my heart. In hindsight, I can say that hormones made those feelings much more dramatic. But it didn't seem that way at the time. Those feelings were real, painful, and overwhelming at times.

Depending on how you look at it, it was either fortunate or unfortunate that I couldn't afford to extend my maternity leave and that I had commitments to patients, interns, and colleagues that I didn't want to break. Forcing myself through that separation was tough, but it was the right thing to do. My anxiety and sadness were real, and I felt them acutely. But they were leading me astray. I needed to get back to my career and get down to the business of settling into the working-parent juggle. If I had listened to those feelings too closely, I would have given up on something I truly loved, something that makes me a better parent.

Prior to having children, I had always thought I would hire a nanny to care for my kids when I returned to work. The cultural bias around day care is quite strong: it seemed that the only reason to choose day care was that it was more affordable than a nanny. But when I started working at the VA hospital in Manhattan, several of my colleagues were taking their babies to the day-care center in the building. I realized that day care was a real option and, when done well, could be the better option.

Day Care or Nanny?

Parents often worry about how child care, whether day care or a nanny, will affect their child's sleep. If their baby is sleeping well, they worry that the shift to child care will derail their gains. And sleep-deprived parents worry that things will get worse. But child care in general is a good thing. Thinking ahead about sleep will ensure a better fit for your baby's and your family's needs. But there are also a lot of other factors to consider when selecting a child-care provider.

Day care often gets short shrift in the conversation about child care because it is less expensive than hiring a nanny. Parents want the best for their kids and reflexively think that the more expensive, one-on-one care of a nanny is superior. There are many advantages to a private nanny or childminder, but there are significant advantages to day care as well. Full disclosure: both of my children went to day care 4–5 full days per week from the age of 4 months.

Benefits of Day Care

A TEAM TAKING CARE OF YOUR BABY. Think about how you feel after a long day alone with your baby. You're tired and you need a break. It's wonderful, of course, but it's also monotonous. Day-care centers have multiple caregivers. If one needs a break, there's someone else to step in. If one is getting frustrated because a baby keeps throwing food on the floor, she can switch places with someone else who has more patience for that task at that particular moment. If one gets sick, there's a sub to be called. Day-care caregivers take care of one another.

THEY WILL PUT YOUR CHILD ON A SCHEDULE. Nannies do this, too, so it's not really an exclusively day-care pro, but it's worth mentioning. Day cares must operate using a system. They serve meals at certain times, have activities at certain times, and put children down to nap at certain times. If you have struggled to get your baby on a schedule, the structure of day care will get it done. Whether it's because your baby is less inclined to fight to stay awake if it's not you putting him down, or it's because the caregiver is calmer and less emotionally invested in whether your child sleeps, babies often nap better when someone other than a parent is putting them down. And then there's the value of peer pressure. As they become more aware of their surroundings, being in a room full of sleeping babies will encourage your baby to join in.

You don't have to be someone's boss. This was a big selling point for me. I just didn't want to manage a business relationship with a nanny. With day care, you accept the terms of their system, and their system works. Of course they must be open to your (reasonable) requests. But you do not have to come up with a contract, manage disagreements, or communicate your parenting style for someone else to emulate.

You won't be jealous of the day-care providers. Parents are often jealous of their child's relationship with the nanny even though they also know how lucky they are to have such a wonderful caregiver. The relationship between your child and day-care providers will be special (my children and I still visit our old day care to say hello), but it does not mimic the parent-child relationship.

Licensed day care is "on the books." A legal contract is better for workers and allows you to claim benefits for child-care expenses. Paying a nanny off the books is very common, but it is risky on many levels. Aside from breaking the law and ruining your chances of ever being elected to public office, employing someone off the books puts you at risk in cases of personal injury and potential payment or contract disputes. It does not exempt you from responsibility for unemployment benefits. Paying a nanny on the books is safer and ethically responsible, but it is also expensive and more complicated.

YOU CAN FOCUS ON DOING YOUR JOB WHEN YOU ARE AT WORK. Being a working parent is hard. You simply have too many things to think about. It's common for nannies to be in touch with parents throughout the day to give updates or ask questions. That seems like a nice idea, until you're in a meeting and your nanny is texting you. It's bad for your job performance, and it keeps you feeling pulled in too many directions. Your day care will call you when there is an urgent concern about your child's health or well-being. Otherwise, you do your job and they do theirs.

YOU DON'T HAVE TO BUY ALL OF THE BIG TOYS. In New York City in particular, this is a huge selling point. Most people don't have playrooms or "bonus rooms" here, and every giant piece of plastic that entertains or teaches your baby takes up valuable space. Your baby is going to be well entertained at day care with a variety of exersaucers, play gyms, and play houses. You will be able to get away with having much less of that at home.

YOUR BABY WILL MAKE FRIENDS, AND YOU PROBABLY WILL, TOO. Your baby will start to recognize the other babies at day care; they form relationships very early. They won't play together with a toy at 6 months old, but they'll sit next to each other in high chairs and "chat" while they eat breakfast. They'll get excited when they see each other. As time goes on, they will develop a strong sense of empathy as well. There's a real comfort and bond among babies who go to day care together. These are their oldest friends, and they often maintain an easy rapport that's like family. It's also an opportunity to meet other parents doing the same juggle, and it's comforting to see others as frazzled as you are (or at least as frazzled as I was) at the end of the day.

THE ACTIVITIES AND CLASSES ARE ON-SITE. Your baby will enjoy an array of activities, such as music, movement, arts and crafts, even yoga, and you won't have to arrange it, pay extra for it, or feel frustrated when your baby sleeps through the activity. This also means that you won't have to cram these "essentials" into your weekends.

You won't have to apply for preschool. Day cares aren't just about child care anymore. There's a real trend toward competing with preschool while still functioning as a working-parent's resource. Preschools tend to have shorter days, some as short as 2 hours. That is not a source of child care for working parents. Day care can provide your child with a preschool structure on a workday schedule with plenty of unstructured playtime mixed in. Your child will learn her letters, numbers, animals, and the canon of pre-school books and songs. She will learn how to sit in a circle, nap on a mat, and eat at a little table with her friends. You won't have to stand in line in the middle of the night for an application or submit to a toddler interview to get in.

Your child will learn how to be dropped off in capable hands (and you will learn how to leave). This is incredibly important. If your baby starts day care before 6 months, separation anxiety will be less of an issue. Babies develop separation anxiety around 6 months. If they are already settled in day care, that process is less intense. Your baby might still cling to you or cry when you leave, but it will be easier for him to settle down when you go. Even if you start your baby in day care after he is 6 months old, getting through the separation process at this age can smooth out more challenging separations that come later on. Day care teaches your child that other people can take care of him and keep him safe. When you walk into your child's nursery class in a few years, he won't understand why you have to stay to help him settle in; he'll be used to doing that for himself.

Disadvantages of Day Care

YOU DON'T HAVE ULTIMATE CONTROL. As I said earlier, this was not a disadvantage for me. I rather liked not having to make every decision about my child's day. But you do have to be willing to join the day care's system, and that might not be your style. If you want to have detailed input into much of your child's day, you might be frustrated by day care. Day cares vary in how involved they want parents to be, so ask around to find a good fit.

THEY PROBABLY WON'T LET YOUR BABY CRY HIMSELF TO SLEEP. After all, there are several babies sleeping in a room at once, and they can't let one wake all of the others. But, in my experience, both personal and professional, babies tend to know that they can get rocked at day care and not at home. They are able to differentiate at a very young age. If it becomes a problem, you can always talk to your day-care provider about making a temporary arrangement for letting your baby cry to teach her to fall asleep independently at day care.

YOUR BABY WILL GET SICK, AND SO WILL YOU. This is a tough one. Babies in day care pick up a lot of colds and viruses no matter what the day care does to sanitize. It's awful when your baby is sick, and it can be very disruptive to everyone. However, it's now or later. And babies who go to day care tend to build stronger immune systems and miss fewer days of primary school than babies who are cared for at home. Your immune system will also bolster itself eventually, and you won't catch everything they bring home.

WHEN YOUR BABY IS SICK, YOU WILL SCRAMBLE. A nanny can come to your home to take care of your baby when she is sick. But you can't send a sick baby to day care. If you don't have family members who can pitch in or some other available backup, it is incredibly stressful to find coverage in a pinch. Fortunately, as day care becomes more popular, emergency babysitting services are springing up, too.

YOU HAVE TO GET YOUR BABY OUT OF THE HOUSE EVERY DAY. If you're like me, it's hard enough to get yourself out the door with everything you need. Add another person to that—one who needs nappies, bottles, and food—and mornings can become a circus.

THE SCHEDULE CAN BE RIGID. This is changing, but most day cares still have a fairly rigid schedule of drop-off and pickup times. If you need very early drop-offs or late pickups, it might not work for you.

YOUR BABY WILL NOT HAVE ONE-TO-ONE ATTENTION ALL THE TIME. I'm including this here because some people think that's a problem. I don't agree. I think it's great for kids to share caregivers. They learn to self-soothe, to be happy alone (under supervision), to wait their turn. However, some parents feel strongly that the one-to-one attention of a nanny is a priority.

Benefits of Hiring a Nanny

YOUR LIFE WILL BE MUCH LESS HECTIC. You set the schedule and design the scope of work to meet your needs. You might still be racing to get out of the house in the morning and to get home at night, but you don't have to do everything yourself. Your nanny will arrive in the morning and take over so you can get going. And she or he might feed and/or bathe your child so you won't have to scramble when you get home.

YOUR BABY WILL HAVE ONE-TO-ONE ATTENTION. Your nanny's attention won't be divided among other kids, which leaves more time for one-to-one interaction. Your baby will get to know her caregiver and rely on her.

YOU SET THE AGENDA. If you have a specific child-rearing philosophy, you can employ your nanny to put it into practice. You can decide whether and how much your child will go to organized activities. You can also decide which children you do or don't want your child to be around.

YOU WON'T GET STUCK WHEN YOUR BABY IS SICK. If your baby is very ill, you want to be with him. But your nanny can take care of things when the crisis is over. You won't have to stay home for every fever, ear infection, or outbreak of conjunctivitus.

YOU WILL KNOW WHAT YOUR BABY DOES ALL DAY. Day-care providers give you a general sense of what happens during the day and a specific report of the essentials (eat, sleep, poop). Your nanny can give you as much or as little information as you want.

Disadvantages of Hiring a Nanny

YOU ARE IN CHARGE. This is not a disadvantage for everyone, but it was the deciding point for me. I was in charge of enough and didn't want more responsibility. When you are the boss, you have to give structure, handle disagreements, and provide feedback. You also have to handle payment, pay rises, holidays, and the occasional personal crisis.

YOU MIGHT BE JEALOUS. Logically, you will know that it is a good thing for your baby and her caregiver to love each other. But you still might be envious of their bond. This can create tension in your relationship with your nanny.

THE NANNY MIGHT LEAVE. Your baby will become attached to her nanny, but your caregiver is not obligated to be part of your family forever. Eventually, your nanny will leave, or you won't need her services in the same way. Handling these transitions can be challenging both emotionally and practically.

NANNIES GET BORED AND FEEL ISOLATED JUST LIKE EVERYONE DOES. Taking care of an infant all day can be monotonous, even for those who adore babies. These days, mobile phones provide a relief and distraction throughout the day with games, calls, and texts. That is helpful on the one hand, but it also takes attention away from your baby. It's important to be explicit up front about your expectations concerning mobile phones, television, and socializing. Handled correctly, those distractions can provide relief that helps keep your nanny engaged.

What to Look For in a Day Care

BEYOND SAFETY, CONVENIENCE, AND REPUTATION. There are plenty of resources available to guide your search for a good day-care center. Obviously, you must make sure the facility is licensed and insured, exceeds required safety practices, and has a clean record with the council and Ofsted. You will also consider your schedule and commute, really thinking through the logistics of your daily life to make sure you won't be running yourself ragged. And you will talk to other parents about their experiences with the day care.

When it comes to sleep, there are a few more things to consider. Keep in mind that, by enrolling your baby in a day care, you are accepting their policies and procedures. You need to make sure that your (sleep) priorities match up with theirs.

WHERE DO THE BABIES SLEEP? This is a big one. Day-care centers that house infants should have a sleeping area separate from the activity area. Your baby is not going to sleep well in a portable cot set up in the corner of a room where other kids are playing, especially if there are older babies or toddlers in the group. A separate, dark, quiet, bedroom-type area makes all the difference when it comes to getting good naps at day care. The bedroom will have multiple cots. Single occupancy is not a requirement (nor is it realistic).

Once your baby is down to a single-nap schedule, a separate sleeping area is not necessary. Toddlers in day care tend to nap all together at the same time on mats. You might think it would be impossible to get a group of toddlers settled down together like that, but somehow it works.

WHEN DO THE BABIES SLEEP? Flexibility of schedule is important. By the time your baby is in day care, she will likely have at least a rough daily sleep schedule. But babies need some flexibility as well. If the schedule at day care is too rigid, your baby might get overtired before nap time and protest or wake up too early. You should feel comfortable walking into your day care at drop-off and telling the caregiver that your baby woke up a little early and might need to go down for the morning nap sooner than usual. Having a separate sleeping space within the day care makes it possible to be flexible.

WILL YOUR BABY HAVE TO DROP A NAP TOO SOON? Some day cares promote babies to an older group when they reach 1 year of age. This is not a problem in and of itself. However, this promotion often coincides with a more rigid, single-nap schedule. If your baby still needs two naps, this could cause some trouble. Dropping the nap prematurely can result in shorter naps, overfatigue, bedtime protests, night waking, or early waking. You might be able to compensate with a very early bedtime (think 6 p.m. or even 5:30), but that is probably going to be hard to manage if your child is in day care in the first place. Find out whether your child will still be able to get a second nap if she needs it. If possible, find a day care that allows a bit more flexibility until a child is 18 months.

IS THERE PRIVATE OUTDOOR SPACE? Why would outdoor space matter for sleep? Imagine trying to get ten babies outside all at the same time. It's quite a feat. A day care with private outdoor space can bring the kids outside a few at a time. That allows the sleeping babies to stay sleeping in the bedroom (with supervision) while others get some fresh air and outdoor activity. Fresh air and sunlight help to set the body clock and keep your baby on the age-appropriate schedule.

Talking to Your Nanny About Sleep

You make the rules when you have a nanny, so it's important to be clear about your expectations and priorities
from the start. During the interview process, ask the
candidates about their views on sleep and their prior
experience. Ask former employers about sleep when
checking references. Before hiring someone, make sure
that he or she will be willing to have the baby nap at
home most of the time and spend most outdoor time
awake. Make sure that your nanny will be comfortable
allowing your baby to fuss or cry at nap times if you ask
him or her to do so. And ask your nanny to keep track
of your baby's sleep during the day. It's important to
know how the day went so you can adjust the bedtime if
necessary.

And Now, Take the Leap

Separating from your baby is a hard process, but so
important to master. If you are anxious about leaving
your baby with a caregiver and you avoid doing it, your
anxiety will intensify. You can come up with endless
excuses to put it off, but you will have to get used to
some version of child care sooner or later. Try to separate your own feelings about this from what your baby

is experiencing. Your baby will be well cared-for with a skilled nanny, childminder or day-care provider. Now take a deep breath and take the leap.

Key Points from Chapter 8

- Leaving your baby in another person's care can be stressful at first, but it's an important milestone for everyone.
- There are pros and cons to all child-care options. The challenge is to find a good fit for your family's needs.
- Thinking ahead about sleep in a child-care setting, either with a nanny or at a day-care center, can save a lot of headaches.
- Look for a day care that understands and prioritizes sleep, providing a separate sleep area for babies as well as a schedule with enough flexibility to accommodate your child's needs.
- When interviewing nannies, discuss their experience and philosophy in relation to sleep. Be clear about your child's needs and make sure that the person you choose understands your expectations about sleep.

CHAPTER 9

Reality Check

Parents often ask if I offer a guarantee that my plan will work. Of course, it makes sense that they would want some sort of reassurance that investing their time, money, and effort will yield results. But guarantees aren't possible in this type of work. We are, after all, working with a human being, not a chemistry set. There are no guarantees because you (and I) can't control all of the factors at play. The baby's temperament; medical or developmental concerns; the parents' anxiety about change, crying, and distress; the parents' level of agreement on priorities around sleep—all of these things affect how the baby settles into a good sleep rhythm.

It's also important to realize that good sleepers aren't 100 percent reliable. They hit bumps like everyone else.

The goal is always to get your baby settled into a good rhythm so that you and your baby can manage and rebound from the curveballs that come your way.

You Can't Control Everything

Parents are often unprepared for the level of chaos that comes with having children. It takes time to develop rhythms and routines, to learn how to parent *your* baby. Kids are messy, unpredictable, and *needy*. They don't fit neatly into your life. Learning to live with less control can be a challenge, but it's a healthy one.

There are two types of control-oriented parents. There are those who need the baby to conform to their schedule and those who orient their entire lives around the baby. Of course, these are the extremes. There are all sorts of variations across the spectrum of control.

MAKING ROOM IN YOUR SCHEDULE FOR THE BABY. Parents who need the baby to conform to their own schedule are not necessarily the hard-driving, narcissistic, out-of-touch type. In fact, most of the parents I meet who are desperate for the baby to be on their schedule are very involved, very loving, and want to spend as much time as possible with their child. They simply have work, financial, or other constraints that are inflexible, making them feel trapped between their obligations and their vision of what parenthood "should" be.

I empathize with these parents. After all, I've been in their shoes. It's hard to take a step back and really look at the way you live your life. You have to acknowledge some tough truths because there's probably a pretty big gap between the way things are going and the way you want them to be. But facing those facts allows you to sort out the things that can't ever change, those that can't change now, those that can change a little, and those that can change a lot. You don't have to turn your whole life upside down to find a better balance.

When you feel boxed in by all of the intractable demands in your life, don't try to find the ultimate solution; fix the sleep first. Do what you have to do to get your child onto a schedule that allows him to sleep well. Then figure out how all of the pieces of your life can fit together to maintain some kind of balance.

Perhaps there are some short-term solutions like flexitime that will allow you to stagger your schedule and get home earlier on some nights. Perhaps you can strike an agreement to work at home a night or two each week after your baby is asleep. Maybe you and your partner can alternate and come home earlier on some nights. Or maybe you'll find that you can stretch your baby's bedtime a couple of nights a week without compromising her sleep. But once you see how happy your baby is when she is sleeping well, it will be easier to tolerate losing a little time with her so she can continue getting the sleep she needs.

MAKING ROOM IN THE BABY'S SCHEDULE FOR YOU. At the opposite extreme are the parents who rely too heavily on the schedule, planning everything to the minute to allow for rigid adherence to routines. These parents are driven by the belief that everything will fall apart if the baby doesn't sleep well *all the time.*

This all-or-nothing thinking—either the baby sleeps well all the time or she is a "bad sleeper"—is a real problem. Even the most reliable sleepers struggle at times. If you pin your self-esteem or your mood on how your child sleeps each day, you are likely to be disappointed. Yes, your life is easier and more pleasant when your baby is not overtired, but you can't achieve this 100 percent of the time. It's normal to feel desperate to maintain the progress you have made after a long haul of sleep deprivation. But a microfocus on sleep schedules is exhausting and unnecessarily restrictive. Once your baby is sleeping reasonably well, shift your focus to the macro-level.

Your baby can tolerate occasional changes to the schedule and routine. You can't possibly plan your whole life around the baby's schedule indefinitely. There will be times when you want or have to be out or cut a nap short or skip one altogether. Your baby won't necessarily be happy about it, but you can get through the fussiness when it's not happening all the time.

You cannot control your baby's demeanor at all times. By teaching your child to sleep and prioritizing sleep in her schedule, you are giving her a solid baseline. Most of the time, she will be rested, and that makes her easier to parent. Although your goal is to keep her well rested and avoid overfatigue, you must also be able to handle the odd times when she is cranky, fussy, and hard to please. If you live in fear of those times, you risk becoming unnecessarily rigid and robbing your family of important experiences like travel, outings, and social gatherings.

You Do Need to Have Some Control

Going with the flow has its advantages, but babies need a good deal of structure to be good sleepers. It should be clear by now that most babies don't settle into a good sleep rhythm without some help from their parents. Sitting back and waiting for your baby to fall asleep or indicate that she's ready to sleep will often result in an overtired and unhappy baby.

There are plenty of things that you can and should

control: bedtime should be early; good naps should be a priority; the routine should be soothing; the baby should then learn to self-soothe. But there are also things that you can't control: teething, your work schedule, illness, neighbors. These things are the normal tricky parts of life, and it's best to learn to roll with them. The happy medium is a schedule with some flexibility that is based upon the baby's biorhythm and need for sleep.

Sleep Is Not Always Perfectly Predictable

When you are in the thick of sleep training, it's important to keep close track of each day's sleep. That kind of focus helps you to figure out where and how your baby is getting overtired and will guide your intervention. But once your baby is sleeping well, you can relax your focus and take a broader view.

Too much focus on each aspect of the schedule will drive you and everyone around you crazy. Your baby will have a basic schedule, but there will be a fair amount of variability day to day. You might have a baby who gets a certain amount of sleep over the course of the three naps but the distribution of that sleep is not very predictable. Some days, the morning nap is long, and the two others are shorter. Other days, there's another configuration. Or you might know that there's a particular "nap-time window" that varies based on factors like the previous nap, activity level, and nighttime sleep. If you remain rigidly fixated on military-like timing, you might be frustrated because your baby does not respond with absolute consistency. Learning to roll with normal variability is important for everyone.

After all, think about yourself: You might not go to bed at the exact same time each night, or it might take you varying amounts of time to fall asleep. Your energy level during the day varies based on a lot of uncontrollable factors, such as season, stress, weather, even pollen count, and not just on how well you slept the night before. If you rely on absolutes when it comes to your baby's schedule, you will feel out of control a lot of the time.

Please remember: Your child is going to blow a nap once in a while, and everything will be all right. There will be days when everything is harder. There will be nights, even strings of nights, when your baby wakes up. These retreats do not signal a collapse of the system, and they do not have to spoil your whole day or week. Remind yourself that babies are constantly growing and changing. You know how to do a quick reboot if it turns out that you really have a problem. But, in most cases, a blip comes and goes as long as you don't reinforce it with heroic efforts to "help."

A bad nap or night doesn't have to ruin your day. You probably know whether it's better to keep your baby active or tone things down when he's having an "off" day. Don't assume that the best thing is to cancel everything and stay home with a grumpy baby. Distraction might very well be best for both of you, even if you're both a little fussy.

Good Sleepers Make Noise During the Night

The goal of sleep training is to teach your baby how to fall asleep and return to sleep independently throughout the night. Your baby might very well cry out from time to time or even cry for several minutes. Because your baby goes through multiple sleep cycles during the night, he might wake fully at some point. Video monitors have created a lot of anxiety because parents (who stay awake to watch) realize that their babies are awake much more than they thought normal. **The problem is not that the baby is awake; it is that the parent is aware of it and treats it as an issue.**

Night waking without prolonged, forceful crying is common. And occasional episodes of longer, more forceful crying are also normal. Instead of thinking, "I'm glad that's over!" when your baby finally becomes a good sleeper, think, "I'm so glad I know how to do this!" You have gained invaluable knowledge and parenting skills through this experience. Of course you don't want to lose ground and repeat sleep training. But you know what to do, what to expect, and most important, why and how the process works. You might have to repeat some crying from time to time, but you and your baby will be better at it each time.

Taking a Step Back

If you find yourself thinking about your baby's sleep schedule most of the time, getting anxious when there will be a schedule disruption, or avoiding all activities that might push your baby even a little bit past nap or bedtime, it's time to step back and get a more objective view.

Start by keeping a sleep diary for a week or two. A simple record of the schedule—whether there is crying, fussing, or night waking—will help you to see how well you are doing. When you look at a sleep diary, you can see how the good measures up against the less good (try not to think of it as the bad). It's easier to battle all-or-nothing thinking this way. You'll see whether things are as unstable as they feel. If they are, it's time to figure out why. But it's often too easy to focus selectively on the harder days or nights, ignoring all of the progress.

While you are assessing your baby's sleep over time, think about your own expectations. If you define success as having a baby who falls asleep without a peep, is silent throughout the night, and wakes up no earlier than 7:30 a.m., you are likely to be disappointed. You can have a fantasy—and it might even be fulfilled occasionally—but it's very important to have realistic expectations so you can know when it's time to stop thinking about sleep as a problem.

Key Points from Chapter 9

- Babies don't just get the sleep they need. Parents have to teach babies how to sleep and provide enough structure to keep them well rested.
- When babies follow a schedule in sync with their biorhythm, it is easier for them to get the restful sleep that they need.
- However, the schedule is not timed to the minute. Sleep times can and will vary somewhat (roughly plus or minus a half hour).
- Finding a balance between structure and flexibility allows your baby to thrive and you to enjoy your time together.
- Everyone wakes up during the night. It is normal to hear your baby during the night from time to time.

Sleeping through the night means that your baby is able to return to sleep independently during normal nighttime arousals.

- Good sleepers aren't perfect every night, but they are well rested overall and flexible enough to rebound from life's curveballs.

CHAPTER 10

When the Baby Is Sleeping but the Parents Aren't

My goal in this book is to give you the information and strategies that you need to get your baby into a healthy sleep rhythm so that you can relax into your new life as a family. If you can count on your baby sleeping, you won't be spending your days—and nights—putting out fires. Your life will start to resemble more of what you thought the joys of parenthood would be.

But what if your own sleep becomes a problem? It's actually very common for new parents to struggle to return to a normal sleep schedule after their baby has learned to sleep through the night. And it's hard to enjoy parenthood when you're exhausted and depleted. Pregnancy, childbirth, postnatal hormonal fluctuations, multiple night feedings or wakings with a newborn,

The adult body clock functions differently from an infant's. Babies and children—even teenagers—need more sleep than adults. The average adult needs between 7 and 8½ hours of sleep. And it's best if that sleep is consolidated into one long chunk at night instead of being broken up into naps and shorter nighttime sleep. Napping, especially more than 20–30 minutes, disrupts nighttime sleep in adults, the exact *opposite* of its effect in babies and toddlers.

weaning—there have been countless causes of sleep disruption in your life in the recent past. Sometimes it takes some work to bounce back.

Things have changed. Your body clock is out of sync. You still listen for your baby, prepared to leap up at a moment's notice even though your baby rarely needs you at night. You might be struggling with hormonal and/or mood fluctuations. The responsibility of parenthood could be heightening your anxiety. Whether you always had trouble sleeping or completely took good sleep for granted, you have a new set of challenges to deal with. You can adjust and learn to sleep well in these new circumstances by taking a good look at your habits and the little things that undermine your sleep. This chapter will help you to understand what's getting in the way of your sleep and give you strategies to get your nights—and days—back into a good rhythm.

Having a Baby Is Stressful, Even When Things Go Smoothly

Let's face it: having a baby is a lot of work. Whether you're over the moon or struggling with postnatal depression, bringing a baby into your life creates stress. And the rest of the stress in your life doesn't just evaporate. Your whole world has been rocked.

By the time you're reading this chapter, you're probably coming up for air after a period of extreme stress and sleeplessness and a crash course in parenthood. You are beginning to find some sort of rhythm to your days and some version of a system for getting things done. You might be back at work already or preparing to return. Or you're getting accustomed to parenting full-time. You've probably been last on your own list for a while now, and it is taking a toll.

Plus the stakes in your life are higher now. There's a human being who is completely dependent on you. It is your job to take care of her physical and emotional needs. She's expensive, too. This new level of responsibility requires a big chunk of your mental energy, and it creates anxiety. There's often an urge to plan out the next phases of your life (career, housing, finances, more babies) as you try to think ahead to when things will finally *calm down*.

Taking Care of Yourself in Increments

There's no magical answer here. In fact, waiting for everything to settle down or fall into place will often just increase your stress level. It's time to put just a little more focus on taking care of yourself. I know it feels like you don't have time, but you do.

The trick is to be realistic. Don't think about the overall picture or set long-term goals right now. This isn't about the 10 kg you still want to lose. It's about carving out 20 minutes to take a brisk walk. It's about letting yourself indulge in gossip magazines or stupid TV—*and feeling good about it*. It doesn't work if you feel like you're wasting time that could be better spent doing laundry. The laundry will get done or it won't. But you need a few minutes to take a real break.

There is value in the incremental. It will make you feel better.

Examples of Incremental Self-Care:

- Get dressed! You might not think it makes a difference, but wearing leggings or PJs all day will start to make you feel exhausted, run-down, and schlumpy.
- Bathe: shower or bath (I call it hydrotherapy). You will feel better.

- Schedule some clothes shopping. You need some real clothes even if you haven't met your goal weight. If you're unhappy with your postnatal appearance, bring a friend or shop online and try things on at home with a supportive partner.
- Take a brisk walk.
- Meet with a friend for coffee or a (gasp!) glass of wine.
- Work through an entire TV series on Netflix. You'll look forward to your daily installment.
- Write in a journal.
- Read a magazine or novel.
- Have a cup of tea.
- Talk on the phone to someone who makes you laugh or calms you, not to someone to whom you feel obligated.
- Other ideas: go for a 10-minute massage, get a manicure, see a movie by yourself during nap time, go to the supermarket by yourself.

Where is your baby while you're doing this? Sleeping! Or with your partner, helper, or parent. It's also possible to do some of these things with your baby in a stroller or carrier.

Do not use self-care time to:
- Clean
- Pay bills

- Make lists
- Sort through your baby's clothes, toys, gear, etc.
- Overindulge in sweets or junk food
- Talk to anyone who makes you think about all of the things you need to do

The time spent on this type of self-care is minimal and doesn't compromise your productivity in any meaningful way. In fact, taking breaks will make you *more* productive when you return to your tasks, *as long as* you don't feel guilty about indulging yourself.

LOWERING YOUR STANDARDS. Perfectionism is your enemy here. It won't let you feel good about anything because *good enough* feels like a failure. It's time to give *good enough* another chance. You do not have to be a perfect parent, housekeeper, bookkeeper, fashion plate, lover, grocery shopper, daughter/son, or friend. And let's not forget about your job if you're back at work. You don't have to be perfect at that either. *Good enough* is just that—good enough. There's plenty of time for excellence. Give yourself a break before you run yourself into the ground. You won't always be a new parent.

If you are stressed out about all of the tasks or projects that have to be

> A very wise friend gave me this invaluable advice: **Don't do anything while the baby is asleep that you can do while the baby is awake.**

done, sit down and make a detailed list. Then divide the list into the easy items, the tasks that can be delegated, the essentials, and the wish list. Share these lists with your partner and anyone else who is helpful. Do not share these lists with anyone who is critical of you. Make a plan to knock some quick jobs off of the easy list. Schedule the essentials. The wish list remains on the horizon, but you can now separate buying nappies (essential) from having the carpet steam cleaned (desirable, but it's waited this long already). You will see your priorities more clearly, and you'll be able to accept deferring some things because your resources are limited.

This is really, really important because your to-do list is growing, probably as quickly as your baby. There is always something to do, and you can't do it all in one day. You must find a way to create a sense of accomplishment without crossing off every single item.

GET SOME EXERCISE. This is a tough one if you don't have help. I am purposely separating it from the list of incremental pleasant activities above because not everyone finds exercise so pleasant. However, exercise will lower your stress level, and it can improve your sleep. Exercise releases endorphins, which act as natural stress-relievers and antidepressants.

Finding time, energy, and motivation to exercise is hard when you have a new baby, but it *will* make you feel good if you don't allow too many unrealistic goals to get in the way. If you're determined to lose 10 kg or go to the gym 5 days a week, you will probably feel overwhelmed. And that will make it less likely that you will exercise at all.

Try this: Figure out when and how you will exercise *once*. Not once a day or once a week but once only. After you do that, you will feel better about yourself, and you will get a realistic sense of what it takes to get it done. *Then* you can start to plan exercise into your schedule— slowly. Be realistic about what you can manage. You might have loved your daily swim at 5 a.m. before you had your baby. But that might not be possible, and it also might not bring you the same pleasure it did when you had fewer responsibilities. Once a week is a good place to begin. You can build from there as you settle into a routine again.

KEEP A JOURNAL. For a while, forget about the journal you think you should keep for your baby to look back on later. Write down your own thoughts: the good, the bad, and the very, very ugly. If your head is swimming, your thoughts tend to become circular and fail to get you the sort of resolution you need. Writing (or even dictating) makes those thoughts at least fairly linear, allowing you to make sense of what you are really thinking and feeling. Once you can do that, you can figure out what you need to do about those thoughts. Perhaps you need to vent. Perhaps you need more practical help. Or perhaps you need emotional help. When your thoughts are a jumble, it's hard to find a way out.

Getting the Sleep You Need

Managing your stress level will improve your sleep in both duration and quality. Beyond general stress, your day is filled with threats to your sleep that you don't give much thought to. If your sleep is suffering, step back and assess your whole day. There are some easy fixes that can make a huge difference when it comes to sleep.

UNPLUG. We are constantly looking at some kind of device these days, whether it's for social or business reasons. There are real consequences to being wired this way. First, laptops and handheld screens, such as smartphones and tablets, emit blue light very close to your face. This has been shown to delay the body's release of melatonin, making it harder to fall asleep at bedtime.

Staying active online also creates body tension and a kind of hyperalertness that keeps the mind in an overactive state. Most online time is essentially multitasking, the antithesis of sleep. And the information you take in before bed plants seeds of rumination that can bother you all night. What benefit do you gain from checking your e-mail right before bed? If you respond to e-mail at night, it lets people know that you are available at all hours, encouraging *more* intrusive e-mails. If you don't answer, you spend time thinking about your response, which leads to ruminating and interferes with your sleep. Is it really true that these things can't wait until morning?

Similarly, set a cutoff time in the evening after which you won't text, look at work e-mail, or take care of home-related business like online shopping or bill paying. I advise my patients to get offline at least 2 hours before bed and much earlier if possible. Give yourself back some time in your evening to truly unwind. Watch television. Talk to your partner. Make some eye contact. Maybe even have sex!

Setting boundaries for the intrusions in your life that increase your stress and keep you from unwinding is hard at first. You will have the urge to check your phone or e-mail. You are an addict, after all. It's called a craving. But the more you ignore that urge to check, the easier it becomes.

Believe it or not, television is the least of all evils: it requires less active engagement, and the screen is farther away from your face, limiting the melatonin delay that you get with laptops and handheld screens. I love to watch television at night, so I'm not going to advise any-one to throw out the set. However, there are some impor-tant caveats:

- Don't watch TV in bed.
- Give yourself some time as a buffer between watch-ing TV and going to bed. One hour is a good buffer if you're having trouble sleeping or if you notice that your sleep is not as restful as in the past.
- Don't watch programmes on a tablet or laptop at night.
- Be smart about what you watch at night: perhaps the 10 p.m. news is not the best choice (and cer-tainly avoid distressing shows about awful things happening to babies).

Finally, power down your laptop and leave it *outside the bedroom* with your phone, tablet, and anything else that might draw you back into the day. If you're gasping and thinking this is impossible, you are not alone. It is pretty much the universal first reaction. However, give it some thought. Creating boundaries between work and rest is going to help you get the sleep you need to function at your best *when it is time to work*.

STOP MONITORING YOUR BABY ALL THE TIME. Baby moni-tors, whether audio or video, will disrupt your sleep. They buzz, beep, blink, and encourage you to stay alert while you are sleeping. Initially they might ease your anxiety about being away from your infant at night. But ultimately they create a kind of hypervigilance that interferes with your sleep. You might have to wean yourself gradually by turning the volume way down. When you get rid of it altogether, you will realize that your baby will wake you if she really needs you. Otherwise, there's no reason to stay on alert.

LIMIT CAFFEINE AND ALCOHOL. Caffeine might be helping you through your day, but it can quickly undermine your nights. Even if it does not keep you awake, caffeine will interfere with your sleep quality, preventing you from getting the deep, restorative sleep that makes you feel good the next day. Eliminate all caffeine after 4 p.m. and consider limiting it further if you are feeling really run-down.

Alcohol similarly affects sleep quality by keeping you in lighter sleep. The process of metabolizing alcohol also wakes you up during the night and early in the morning. Alcohol might help you to unwind and feel sleepy, but it isn't really helping your sleep. You don't have to abstain completely, just limit your intake and don't drink too close to bedtime (a minimum of 1 hour, but earlier is better).

You can experiment with changing these habits to determine whether alcohol and caffeine are affecting your sleep. Keep a sleep diary to track your intake during the day, how long it takes you to fall asleep, how many times you wake up in the night, and how rested you feel in the morning. Make one change at a time and allow 3 or 4 days to see a pattern.

"DISCHARGE" THE BUSINESS OF THE DAY. Racing thoughts at bedtime are a common problem among new parents. You have a lot on your mind in many different realms of your life. You are keeping track of a lot, too much for one person. Whether it's staying stocked with nappies, paying bills, juggling work demands, managing friendships and family relationships, or figuring out when you'll get your next haircut (or shower), your mind is understandably overwhelmed. And you're going strong all day without much downtime, so it's easy to be flooded with these to-dos when you first have a chance to relax—at bedtime. The trouble is you can't do anything about any of these to-dos in the middle of the night. So you're stuck making mental lists that you'll probably forget by morning, when the process starts all over again.

But you can get off that hamster wheel, and you don't have to be insanely organized to make it happen. Start by setting aside 15 minutes before your bedtime routine (earlier in the evening is better if you can manage it). Sit down with a pad of sticky notes or a notebook and make some lists. It's a simple solution. Making the time is the hard part. You'll find, though, that this will save you time once you get in the habit of getting these things out of your head (where they will get lost) and onto your refrigerator door (where you or, even better, someone else will pick them up to take care of in the light of day).

As you get into the habit of discharging the business of the day, you can also keep a pad and pen by the bed. When to-dos pop into your head, write them down instead of worrying about whether you'll remember them in the morning. Eventually, you'll get good enough at your evening to-do list ritual that you won't be plagued by those thoughts popping up at bedtime.

DON'T TALK BUSINESS WITH YOUR PARTNER AT BEDTIME. This can be hard because you need to bring each other up to speed on the business of your lives, whether it's work or home-related tasks. But you're tired at night, and it's easy to get frustrated with each other. And you have already made your to-do lists, so don't rekindle all of those racing thoughts. Set aside a time to talk to your partner about essentials. You might be able to do some of it by phone or even e-mail during the day, saving your time together for more pleasant conversation.

ESTABLISH A BEDTIME ROUTINE. You can establish your own sleep cues, just as you have done for your baby. Ever find yourself doing housework until bedtime? Although it's great to wake up to a clean house, you are stressing yourself out before bed. You need a routine to help you unwind, to separate your day from your night.

Your routine does not have to be elaborate. It might include just getting dressed for bed, washing up, and reading for 15–20 minutes. If you need more to help you unwind, take a shower or bath, do a relaxation exercise, or do some simple stretching to release body tension. The key is to give yourself a buffer between your (over)active day and bedtime.

READ FICTION. Reading fiction is great for sleep as long as you are not reading an e-reader with a backlight (low-tech e-readers without a backlight are fine). Reading provides an escape. You are focused on the story, creating your own images as you read the text. This occupies your mind, diverting it from all of the other mental clutter from the day. Without all of that rumination, your body will relax, and you will get sleepy. Over time, reading will become a sleep cue that actually induces sleepiness. That can be frustrating when you can't stay awake long enough to get through a chapter, but you could have much worse problems.

If you find that you wake up for prolonged periods during the night, read some more. The distraction and physical effort fatiguing your eyes will help you return to sleep without the frustration and adrenaline release that can be triggered by night-waking insomnia. It's best to read using a small lamp or book light. Try to avoid turning on overhead lights as this can be disruptive to your body's sleep clock.

Again, use your judgment about content. If you get too excited, sad, or scared reading certain genres, avoid them. It's a great time to re-read old classics that carry you away without being too taxing.

RELAXATION EXERCISES. Most people who have trouble sleeping tell me that relaxation exercises don't help them. But most of those people are misusing the exercises. If you do a relaxation exercise expecting to fall asleep, your anxiety will mount. As you get further into the exercise, you will become frustrated that it's not working, and your body will respond with adrenaline. However, if you use a relaxation exercise for its intended purpose—relaxation—it can be very helpful. Forget about falling asleep. The point is to prepare your body for sleep, to clear your mind, slow down your heart rate and respiration, and release body tension. If you stop pressuring yourself to sleep on cue, you'll relax, and then you'll fall asleep more easily.

The kind of relaxation exercise you use is up to you. You can buy or download guided relaxation of all varieties. Try a few during the day when you're not stressed out. Find a couple of recordings that you like, with narrators whose voices are soothing. Practice when you are feeling good, at least once a day for several days. This will train your body to associate the exercise with relaxation, heightening its benefit. Once you have learned to relax with the exercise under optimal conditions, you can start trying it out at bedtime. But remember: This is a relaxation aid, not a sleep aid.

Resetting Your Body Clock

New parents throw out all of the rules for good sleep hygiene because they have to. You can't always go to bed at the same time every night, and your nights have been disrupted by your baby. It doesn't make sense to get up at a set wake-up time in the morning if you don't have to. And you might be napping, too. You need all the sleep you can get.

When you are sleep deprived and focused solely on the baby's development, it's acceptable—and perhaps unavoidable—to let your own healthy sleep habits slide. Now that your baby is sleeping, it's time to get yourself back into a good sleep rhythm. The easiest way to set your body clock is to set your alarm and get up at the same time every day. A consistent wake-up time will lead to a consistent bedtime. Will you ever be able to sleep late when you have the opportunity? Yes. But just as you put your baby through sleep boot camp to establish good habits, you need to do the same for yourself. Be a purist for a week or two to allow your body to get back on track.

If you are having trouble sleeping at night, don't nap. I know this might sound awful. But nighttime sleep is the priority. Once you are sleeping well at night, you can experiment with naps of different lengths and at different times to see whether there are ways to nap without compromising your nights.

Remember: The rules are different for adults. Babies and toddlers sleep better when they are *less* tired, so making up for lost sleep will help them. But adults need less sleep, and so a healthy amount of fatigue helps us to fall asleep quickly and lessens nighttime interruptions.

The idea here is to produce some fatigue so that you can go to bed at a normal time, fall asleep easily, and sleep until morning with minimal, if any, night waking. If you are constantly making up for lost sleep by napping during the day or sleeping late in the morning, your body won't be able to return to a normal schedule at night. You have to let yourself be tired and avoid compensating for lost sleep. Your body will recalibrate itself if you stop interfering.

DON'T GO TO BED TOO EARLY. Jumping into bed at 8 p.m. isn't going to help you if you're not sleepy. And, realistically, you don't need 12 or even 10 hours of sleep. Going to bed early and "trying" to sleep will actually make your problem worse. The more time you spend in bed awake and frustrated, the more difficult it will be to fall asleep. Your body releases adrenaline when you are frustrated, and it will take you longer to calm down and fall asleep. Repeated frustration at bedtime will also lead to a kind of performance anxiety as bedtime approaches. If you get anxious in the evenings, expecting to have a rough time falling asleep, you will create a self-fulfilling prophecy. That anxiety assures that you *will* have trouble falling asleep.

DON'T WORRY ABOUT WAKING DURING THE NIGHT. We all wake up during the night as we transition out of one sleep cycle and into another. Most of the time, we aren't aware of waking and might just roll over or let out a big sigh. But it is also normal to be aware of waking up during the night. As long as you return to sleep fairly easily, brief night waking is not a problem.

You might be more prone to disrupted sleep now because you are used to waking up to take care of your baby. As you get used to your baby sleeping through the night, this should improve. However, if you get upset, angry, or anxious about waking during the night, it will be more difficult to go back to sleep because your body will be full of adrenaline.

To avoid the adrenaline response, try to defuse the situation with some positive self-talk. Remind yourself that it's normal to wake up. Tell yourself that you will be able to go back to sleep even if it takes a little while. Remember that you have been functioning for months with broken sleep, and being awake during the night is not going to kill you, ruin your day, make it impossible to parent, etc. (Remember the earlier discussion of *good enough*?)

Don't use your phone, turn on your computer or tablet, post about insomnia on Facebook, clean, or stay in bed tossing and turning when you are awake during the night. If you are unable to go back to sleep in 15–20 minutes, get out of bed and read until you are sleepy. You can also do a relaxation exercise to help you unwind (but not to fall asleep). Do not go back to bed until you feel you are ready to fall asleep. Do not decide that it's been long enough and you'll just "try." **That won't work.** You will get back to sleep faster if you stay out of bed until you are really ready to sleep. Otherwise your frustration will mount, and you will truly be unable to sleep.

Jennifer: Perfectionism, Guilt, and a Few Bad Habits Create Chronic Insomnia

I first worked with Jennifer when her 4-month-old baby, having suffered from colic, was not rebounding and learning how to get the sleep he needed. Two years later, she contacted me to help her relearn how to sleep. Six months earlier, she had begun struggling to return to sleep in the middle of the night when she would have normal nighttime arousals or wake up to use the bathroom. Now, she was pregnant again and, with increased nighttime trips to the bathroom, the resulting insomnia had become unbearable.

At our first meeting, Jennifer described feeling crippled by insomnia and fatigue. She believed that it was preventing her from being the mother her son deserved. She also believed that it was limiting her productivity at work. Jennifer felt as though she was failing. Beneath the surface was a real struggle with perfectionism. Jennifer believed that she had to do everything perfectly—and feel happy, too.

Jennifer's fatigue made her feel unproductive, and that led to feeling overwhelmed by all of the tasks that were piling up. She found herself ruminating about tasks and making mental lists when she woke up during the night. Thoughts such as "If I don't get the sleep I need, I won't be able to get that report done tomorrow" and "If I don't get more sleep, I'll be cranky, and I won't be the mother my son deserves" were creating more stress and pressure to fall asleep. And the more pressure she put on herself, the more difficult it was to fall asleep.

In addition to her anxiety-producing thoughts, Jennifer had picked up some bad habits along the way. She was going to bed earlier than usual because she was exhausted, but she was starting to have trouble falling asleep at bedtime. She was doing work and shopping for things like nappies on the Internet late into the evening, and she was lying in bed tossing and turning when she couldn't fall asleep.

The first things we worked on were Jennifer's schedule and habits. She set a cutoff time for electronics and started reading in bed until she was very sleepy. We set an earliest bedtime, so she wouldn't be forcing herself to try to catch up on sleep, a strategy that had backfired when she tried it in the past. She began sitting down earlier in the evening, right after putting her son to bed, to think through her to-dos and write them down, in order to preempt the ruminating she had been doing in the middle of the night. The most challenging change was getting out of bed during the night if she wasn't able to return to sleep quickly. She planned to get up and read in the living room, returning to bed when she felt ready to sleep.

The initial changes worked well, and Jennifer immediately began to get more sleep. She rarely had to get out of bed in the middle of the night, as she was able to distract herself and avoid ruminating, which enabled her to return to sleep quickly. She found reading at bedtime to be very soothing and noticed that her sleep seemed to be more restful with the limits on electronics. But she continued to get very frustrated when she had more difficult nights, criticizing herself and predicting worst-case scenarios for the next day.

So we began to work on Jennifer's all-or-nothing thinking. She believed that feeling fatigued was ruinous, that it meant she would be a failure. But Jennifer's standards were so high that they left little room for error. And they were high across the board, in all aspects of her life. For someone to meet those standards in so many different roles would be impossible. And not living up to those standards made Jennifer feel like a failure.

We worked on the concept of "good enough," articulating Jennifer's true priorities and determining areas where relaxing her standards would matter less. She began to do things to make her life easier, like setting up a regular grocery delivery of all of her staples instead of running around to various specialty stores all week long. She could still go to the farmers' market for perfect in-season local strawberries, but she never had to worry about stocking up on nappies or applesauce. We also worked on being kinder to herself about her mothering and her performance at work. Jennifer challenged her belief that she should be happy, energetic, and creative at all times with her son. Understanding the value in imperfection—that her son would see a range of her moods and benefit from not being entertained at all times—

Simple rules of sleep hygiene can improve your sleep dramatically.

1. Get up at the same time each day to set your body clock.
2. Do not try to make up for lost sleep by going to bed early, sleeping later, or napping.
3. Go to bed at roughly the same time each night, but . . .
4. Do not get into bed until you are sleepy.
5. Get out of bed if you are unable to sleep for 15–20 minutes.
6. Create a bedtime routine.
7. Unplug at least 1 hour before bed and keep mobile phones, laptops, and tablets out of the bedroom.
8. Limit caffeine overall and eliminate it after 4 p.m.
9. Limit alcohol close to bedtime.
10. Don't smoke!
11. Limit all fluids for 2 hours before bed.
12. Reserve the bed for sleep, sex, and prebedtime reading.

was freeing for her, although it took some practice to learn to stop criticizing herself.

It took a couple of months, but Jennifer found a healthy sleep rhythm again and stopped getting so stressed out by occasional bad nights. She also learned how to take better care of herself and accommodate the new responsibilities of family life by putting less pressure on herself to be perfect in every way.

SLEEP AIDS. I am not opposed to the use of sleep aids for short-term sleep issues. There are times when medication is the fastest, most reliable solution to a specific situation of sleeplessness. However, sleep aids treat the symptom of sleeplessness. If you have chronic insomnia, sleep aids reinforce feelings of helplessness and performance anxiety. If you find yourself taking sleep aids more than very occasionally, I recommend consulting a psychologist or psychotherapist who specializes in sleep disorders (or at least cognitive behavioral therapy) to treat the underlying causes of insomnia instead of just the symptoms.

Here is some basic information about a few common sleep aids. It is best to consult with your doctor, even if you're taking nonprescription medication and especially if you are breastfeeding. Do not combine sleep aids—prescription, herbal, or over-the-counter—unless prescribed by a medical professional, and do not combine sleep aids with alcohol or drugs.

- Over-the-counter sleep aids (Sominex, Nytol). The only sleep aid approved for sale without prescription is an antihistamine, most commonly Benadryl. Antihistamines can induce drowsiness. These are most effective for occasional use because the drowsiness effect lessens over several days. If you are taking one of these medications, it is best to take it in a formulation that does not include unnecessary analgesics or cold medicine.

- Melatonin: Just because it's "natural" does not mean that it is safe or better than a synthetic or chemical sleep aid. In the UK it is only used to treat insommia in people over the age of 55. Keep in mind that melatonin is a hormone that the body produces naturally. There's no need to supplement this hormone on a regular basis.

- Valerian, chamomile, herbal remedies: Herbal remedies don't hurt, but they don't have a strong effect either. On their own, they are unlikely to have a significant impact on insomnia other than the benefit of their relaxing qualities.

- Prescription hypnotics (Zolpidem): These medications are effective sleep aids available by prescription only. This class of sleep aid is not physically addictive. However, these medications can be psychologically addictive as a person becomes anxious about his or her ability to sleep without them. That anxiety makes it more difficult to sleep and often results in taking medication more often than intended or desired. Used on occasion, these medications can be very helpful. But as with any medication, there can be side effects and they are not recommended if you are breastfeeding.

- Antianxiety medication/benzodiazepines (Lorazepam): These medications treat anxiety and can cause drowsiness. The drowsiness effect lessens over time and the real benefit comes from anxiety relief. However, these medications are physically addictive and the body develops a tolerance for them (meaning you will have to increase your dose over time, and you will have to taper the dose when you are ready to stop). Breastfeeding mothers and those wishing to conceive should always consult their doctor.

Is This Something More? Postnatal depression and/or anxiety can cause insomnia. Most new mums (and dads, too) experience mood fluctuations in the first few months of parenthood. Symptoms can emerge soon after giving birth or even several months later. If you are crying daily, feeling overwhelmed by things big or small, isolating yourself, feeling depressed, anxious, or panicky, talk to someone.

Many women have a hard time judging whether their symptoms are "really" postnatal depression or anxiety. When you are in it, it is very difficult to judge. These experiences aren't shameful, but they *feel* shameful. Women blame themselves for not being good enough or for being naive about birth, newborns, breast-feeding . . . about almost anything. Other new mothers they know seem somehow normal and perfect, having easily adjusted to motherhood and the revolution in their lives.

The trouble is, this is the depression talking. Women who suffer from postnatal mood changes are no worse or better at motherhood than anyone else. They are simply possessed by the hormonal demons that strike a good percentage of new mums. Get treatment, and the clouds will part. You'll see how distorted your judgment was and you'll take back your life.

Don't wait to get help. If you don't know where to begin, ask your GP or midwife for a referral to a therapist and/or psychopharmacologist who is experienced in reproductive psychiatry. **If you are having thoughts about harming yourself, your baby, or anyone else, or if you are experiencing auditory hallucinations (voices talking or mumbling), go to the accident and emergency department at your nearest hospital to get immediate help.**

Dads can experience mood changes as well. Feelings of helplessness, anxiety, fear for the baby's safety, depression over the loss of freedom or increased responsibility—these are just a few examples. Although these symptoms are typically less volatile than they are in a new mother whose hormones are all over the place, they are nonetheless distressing and important to address whether it be with social support (dads' groups) or with therapy or medication.

Take Care of You

One of my first mentors made a habit of saying ". . . and don't forget to take care of *you*" at the end of our meetings. I was volunteering as a teenager at a home for troubled youth, and my mentor knew that the burnout factor was intense. I used to joke about his hokey saying with my friends, but here I am all these years later—let's just say "decades"—repeating it to you.

Parenting is joyful, rewarding, mind-blowing, and fabulous. But it's also exhausting, depleting, unglamorous, and really hard. You can't put yourself last all the time, and you certainly can't do it indefinitely. You'll have to come last sometimes, but please remember that your own health and happiness are worthy investments. And so, dear parents, don't forget to take care of *you*.

Cry-It-Out: Is It Harmful?

Before I became a parent, I was well aware of the divide between those who were attempting so-called attachment parenting and those who were not. After all, I was living in Park Slope, Brooklyn, perhaps the birthplace of helicopter parenting. The divide could often be boiled down to whether a family wanted to cosleep or not and whether they would use crying to "sleep-train" their child. At the time, the argument against crying was centered in the idea that a baby's trust would be violated and the bond with the mother disrupted if the baby were left to cry unattended for any period of time.

In *The Baby Book* (Little, Brown, 1992 and 2003; Hachette Digital, Inc., 2013) and their subsequent publications, William Sears and his coauthors suggest that "night parenting" by responding to babies' every noise fosters secure attachments. But, in my opinion, there are many serious and troubling problems with this doctrine. First and foremost, Dr. Sears is conflating a concept of his own invention, called attachment parenting, with attachment theory.

Attachment theory is the study of the relationship between types of infant-mother attachment and long-term outcomes like personality and emotional adjustment. This theory, backed by a tremendous body of research, is based on the empirical study of the various types of infant attachment and how they relate to personality development. Infants who develop a secure attachment to the parent use him or her as a secure base from which to explore the world. This attachment is accomplished by consistently responding to the baby's needs.

Sears's "attachment parenting" is his philosophy that constant physical closeness (i.e., baby wearing, breast-feeding, and cosleeping) will foster an intense mother-child bond. But "attachment parenting" has not been scientifically demonstrated to form the type of secure attachment that predicts healthy long-term adjustment in the attachment theory literature.

There are several serious problems with Sears's approach. First, babies actually do benefit from being allowed to fuss or cry. A baby whose every whimper results in breastfeeding will not learn other strategies to self-soothe. Second, this method is grueling for parents, who are made to feel guilty or selfish when they are unable to execute it. When it isn't working, parents fear that something is wrong with them or that their bond with their child will be damaged. Sears discusses "night parenting" as something parents must embrace indefinitely. The tone of his philosophy is that parenting must involve complete selflessness. My position is that this utter lack of interpersonal boundaries is psychologically unhealthy for everyone involved.

When it comes to parenting philosophy—or any philosophy for that matter—I respect a person's right to his or her opinion. I disagree with the philosophy of attachment parenting partly because it doesn't feel right to me as a parent and partly because it feels very wrong to me as a psychologist.

Still, as a philosophy it appeals to some parents. If it works for them, I have to respect their personal choice. But somewhere along the line, the message changed from one of bonding to one of real physical harm.

I first heard of this in 2009, when a concerned client asked me my opinion about the scientific literature on crying and brain damage. My first reaction was panic: Had I been unknowingly advising parents to do something harmful? Had I done this awful thing to my own children? But I was trained as a social scientist, and I know how to do a literature search. So I got to work.

It is one thing to suggest that allowing a baby to cry to sleep affects trust, bonding, and attachment. It is quite another to declare that there is scientific proof that cry-it-out can cause brain damage. The first is an opinion, one with which a person is free to agree or disagree. The second is an erroneous assertion of fact that has gone largely unchecked. These are scare tactics, and, in my opinion, they are simply untrue.

There is no scientific literature linking controlled crying or extinction with brain damage or other neurological effects. Unfortunately, one unfounded claim of a scientific link turned into a viral proliferation of erroneous information. Suddenly, "scientists say crying leads to brain damage" was all over the Internet, from message boards to random blogs to *Psychology Today*. But, still, there were no legitimate scientific sources—and there still aren't.

I've been giving a speech about this for more than 5 years to every client, class, and random person at a cocktail party who has the misfortune to ask me what I do for a living. Fortunately, one person who listened happened to be my editor, and she agreed that I should take this opportunity to set the record straight.

"Scientists Say . . ."

The claim that using extinction or crying methods of sleep training can cause physiological damage to babies appears to have originated with Dr. Sears. On his website, Askdrsears.com, there are several references to this "scientific" finding. Others, ranging from mum bloggers to credentialed professionals, have carried on the message, referring to the Sears posts as a main source. The problem is that all of these assertions are based on extrapolation from the published data, which are beyond what can reasonably be presumed. The studies cited simply can't be applied to the claims about the dangers of cry-it-out.

In Sears's often-referred-to post on his website, "Science Says: Excessive Crying Could Be Harmful," the citations simply do not support the claims he makes. What follows here is a step-by-step look at these claims and what can legitimately be inferred from the science.

Sears begins his argument stating: "Research has shown that infants who are routinely separated from their parents in a stressful way have abnormally high levels of the stress hormone cortisol as well as lower growth hormone levels." The impact of this imbalance is, by his interpretation, "inhibit[ion of] the development of nerve tissue in the brain as well as negative effects on growth and the immune system."

To support this statement, he cites studies of rats and monkeys that were manipulated in a laboratory (Butler et al., 1978; Kuhn, 1978; Coe et al., 1985). Certainly, we can learn something from the study of nonhuman babies (particularly primates). These studies suggest that separation from the mother can cause a physical stress response. We know this to be true of sleep training in infants as well. The experience is most certainly stressful and, although studies in this area are limited, there could very well be a physical stress response (i.e., elevated cortisol).

The comparison of human infants to rats and monkeys, however, is limited by the myriad differences in child rearing, cognitive development, psychosocial development, and—to be even more obvious—environment (i.e., indoors, wearing nappies and clothing, etc.). In other words, human babies have needs that are very different from those of infant rats and monkeys. Extrapolating too far from animal laboratory studies of separation leads quickly to inappropriate conjecture.

Sears also cites studies of children undergoing the temporary stress of transitioning to child care (Ahnert et al., 2004). The argument here is that separation from the parent causes increases in cortisol levels *and* that this could be harmful to development. However, the study cited observed 15-month-old children and determined that attachment style (not attachment parenting style) predicted crying during separation and adjustment. Cortisol levels were indeed elevated temporarily during this naturally stressful event. These data suggest—again—that crying and separation during sleep training could also cause a spike in cortisol levels. However, the effect of that spike long term and short term is not determined in this study, despite Sears's implication that such an occurrence is harmful to development. In other words, yes, stress can cause a spike in cortisol, but any discussion of long-term consequences is pure speculation and clinically unfounded.

Next, Sears cites research that persistent or prolonged crying in infancy predicts attention deficit hyperactivity disorder (Wolke et al., 2002), poor emotion regulation (Stifter & Spinrad, 2002), as well as low IQ and deficits in fine motor skills (Rao et al., 2004). A closer examination of these studies clarifies two important reasons why they cannot be applied to the discussion of crying during sleep training. First, the prolonged crying occurred despite the parents' attempts to soothe the child. This type of crying is qualitatively different from the short-term crying used in sleep training. Second, it was the inconsolable aspect of the crying that was of interest to the investigators. These studies were an attempt to understand whether such crying is a symptom of an underlying neurological or developmental issue that could lead to impairments later in childhood, thereby suggesting a course of early treatment intervention. There is no suggestion that the crying itself causes impairments.

Sears also argues that separation and crying can cause "harmful physiologic changes" in infants. Again, the studies cited are not applicable to the use of crying in sleep training. Studies of children with serious illness who are separated from their parents for treatment (Hollenbeck et al., 1980), rat pups separated from their parents (Hofer, 1983; Hofer & Shair, 1982), and neonates in the hospital just days after birth (Brazy, 1988; Ludington-Hoe et al., 2002) are not applicable to the process of teaching a normal, healthy, months-old baby to sleep using cry-it-out.

Finally, Sears uses other study findings to conclude that using cry-it-out causes chemical, functional, and structural changes in the brain. He claims that allowing a baby to cry alone can create an "over-active adrenaline system," resulting in violence, impulsivity, and aggression later on. However, the study cited had nothing to do with cry-it-out. In fact, it examined the effect of chronic exposure to violence (Perry, 1997).

Similarly, Sears cites studies of children exposed to what is called *toxic stress*, or the chronic and overwhelming stress of abuse, neglect, poverty, homelessness, mentally ill caregivers, chronic illness, and the like. He equates cry-it-out with toxic stress and therefore attributes to it the same tragic outcomes. It is true that children who have been raised in institutions, traumatized, and/or neglected suffer from intellectual and social deficits (Lieberman & Zeanah, 1995). It is also true that children exposed to extreme stress demonstrate neurobiological changes (Kaufman & Charney, 2001; Teicher et al., 2003), but one cannot equate cry-it-out with toxic stress.

What the Leading Scientists *Really* Say

Research on Cry-It-Out/Extinction

The scientific literature on extinction-based sleep interventions demonstrates the safety and efficacy of these methods. A task force appointed by the American Academy of Sleep Medicine conducted a rigorous review of studies to determine best practices in the treatment of pediatric sleep disturbance. In 2006, Mindell and colleagues (2006) published the extensive review of 52 studies of sleep interventions in babies and toddlers under 5 years of age. Nineteen of those studies examined unmodified extinction methods used with a total of 552 participants. Another 14 studies (748 participants) examined graduated extinction, better known as the "Ferber method." In all but two of the included studies, the use of extinction methods for sleep interventions resulted in positive outcomes for the child. Furthermore, there were no negative outcomes noted in any of the studies, even those that failed to produce positive outcomes. That's 1,300 babies and no adverse effects. The findings of the task force concluded that extinction methods have the strongest empirical support among interventions to treat sleep disturbance in babies and toddlers. In other words, **top sleep researchers in the United States say that extinction methods are proven to be safe and effective.**

One study of sleep-disturbed infants treated with extinction demonstrated improvement on a scale of sleep behavior, increase in security on an established measure, and potential increases in agreeableness and likability when compared with a control group (France, 1992). Similarly, Eckerberg (2004) found that sleep-disturbed children demonstrated more insecurity before treatment and that insecurity was significantly reduced by the treatment intervention. Furthermore, the more anxious the child prior to the intervention, the greater the emotional benefit of the treatment (Eckerberg, 2004). In their review (which includes the 2004 Eckerberg study), Mindell and colleagues (2006) also noted that there were significant secondary benefits to extinction methods that went along with improved sleep. Several of the reviewed studies noted increases in reported infant security, predictability, irritability, and crying/fussiness. And several of the included studies noted improved parental well-being, stress, and marital satisfaction (Mindell et al., 2006).

In a randomized study of controlled crying in infants age 6–12 months, persistent infant sleep problems predicted higher levels of maternal depression (Hisock & Wake, 2002), which has implications for infant development and attachment (Teti et al., 1995; Martins & Gaffan, 2000). Infants treated with controlled crying had significantly better sleep than that of the control group 2 months after the intervention, but those differences were no longer significant at the 4-month follow-up (Hisock & Wake, 2002). In a follow-up study conducted 5 years posttreatment, there was no evidence of positive or negative consequences of the crying intervention (Price et al., 2012).

The Impact of Sleep Training on Attachment

Research studies simply do not support claims that extinction methods of sleep intervention cause disruptions to parent-infant attachment. Črnčec, Matthey & Nemeth (2010) present a thorough review of the current literature, noting the dearth of studies pointing to a negative relationship between extinction and attachment. They make several key points regarding this claim. First, they note that infant-parent attachment is formed during the day as well as at night, thus using extinction to treat sleep problems does not alter the relationship during the day. Second, they note that parental sleep deprivation and maternal depression associated with infant sleep problems have empirically demonstrated effects on infant attachment, thus implying that teaching a child to sleep improves the quality of daytime parenting. Finally, they found that studies of cultures that promote immediate response to infants' nighttime arousals do not demonstrate healthier infant attachment than cultures that promote extinction-based sleep interventions.

The Truth About Cortisol

Much of the concern about using extinction methods of sleep training comes from a fear of exposing the baby to excessive amounts of cortisol. Cortisol levels fluctuate in the body throughout the day. This process, however, is not well understood in infants. Further, researchers do not have sufficient studies to determine healthy versus unhealthy levels of infant cortisol (Middlemiss et al., 2013). In a longitudinal study of cortisol in infants, De Weerth and van Geert (2002) demonstrated widely fluctuating infant cortisol levels from 5 to 8 months of age, noting that there is no identifiable *normal* level of infant cortisol.

In an often-cited study of infant and mother cortisol response following extinction, Middlemiss and colleagues (2012) measured the salivary cortisol of mothers and infants throughout the process. They found that cortisol was synchronized between mothers and infants on the first day of sleep training. However, by the third day, infants were no longer exhibiting behavioral distress and mothers' cortisol was lowered, but the infants' cortisol remained high. Some critics of extinction methods interpret this as indication of harm incurred during cry-it-out. However, the study ended at day three of sleep training, and there are no data to determine how long cortisol remained elevated or whether such elevations have any significant short- or long-term impact on the baby's development.

Studies indicate that behavioral distress does not necessarily predict the amount of elevation in cortisol (Gunnar et al., 1988). In one study of newborns, behavioral distress was positively correlated with cortisol elevation following circumcision or blood sampling, but the measures of distress were negatively correlated following height and weight check and discharge examination. Furthermore, although soothing with a dummy reduced behavioral distress in babies during a blood sampling and discharge exam, soothing did not reduce cortisol levels (Gunnar et al., 1988). In other words, just because a baby is crying does not mean that cortisol is elevated. Likewise, just because a baby is being soothed does not mean that cortisol is reduced. This is, of course, confusing. But the take-home point is that we cannot assume that an infant is having an adrenocortical stress response (cortisol spike) just because he is crying.

In another study, researchers tracked changes in cortisol reactivity and behavioral distress over time in response to a physical exam with vaccinations. Cortisol reactivity was highest at the 2-month visit and decreased dramatically at the 4-month visit. Notably, this decrease is correlated with increases in sleep between 2 and 4 months of age. Cortisol reactivity decreased dramatically again between the 6-month and 15-month visit. However, behavioral distress *increased* at the 15-month visit (Gunnar et al., 1996). Thus, crying and cortisol are not necessarily correlated.

In a study of 78 healthy infants between 7 and 15 months old, Larson and colleagues (1998) examined cortisol and behavioral reactivity to a mock physical exam. They found that cortisol reactivity to the stressful situation was higher in younger infants. Furthermore, cortisol reactivity largely disappeared by 10–12 weeks of age. However, behavioral distress did not decrease with age (Larson et al., 1998). Once again, the data suggest that we cannot assume that a crying baby is having a physiological stress response.

More research is needed to better understand the role of cortisol in the infant stress response. Extinction methods might very well cause spikes in cortisol levels, although research on cortisol reactivity suggests that this cannot be inferred based on behavioral distress alone. Regardless of whether cortisol is at play, the short-term stress of extinction methods has not been associated with a negative outcome.

What About Long-Term Effects of Cry-It-Out?

To adequately study the long-term effects of cry-it-out, one would have to control for the myriad stressors that could otherwise account for psychological or neuropsychological outcomes later in life. We could

It sounds very scientific to talk about crying causing elevated cortisol. Whether or not crying even does cause cortisol spikes, how can we know what the impact of that particular spike will be? If you are concerned about the impact of the cortisol supposedly caused by cry-it-out, consider it in context. How does several hours of crying spaced out over several nights compare with the physical impact of chronic sleep deprivation—yours and the baby's—over months or years?

measure cortisol levels before, during, and after sleep training, but what would that tell us? We don't know what that specific spike in cortisol would do. Presuming it has some singular effect, a well-designed study would have to measure cortisol response to numerous lifetime stressors and control for those across subjects. If my son cried for 40 minutes during cry-it-out, had to get stitches in his chin at age three, and had ear grommet surgery at age two, how does that compare to your daughter's 2 hours of crying and uneventful medical history?

The point is that there are constant transient stressors in childhood. I consider sleep training to be one of those, but it is a stressor that has a huge positive side. The chronic stress of sleep deprivation—on the child and on the parents—creates a far more disruptive developmental environment both physically and emotionally.

As far as I'm concerned, the long-term effects of cry-it-out are positive. I am not aware of scientific studies that could definitively prove this by following sleep-trained infants into adulthood. But, based on the available pediatric literature as well as my clinical experience with hundreds of babies *and* my knowledge of adult psychopathology, I am convinced. I truly believe that teaching our children to sleep is one of the most valuable lessons in life. Teaching your baby to self-soothe, to understand when her body is tired, to return to sleep during normal nighttime arousals, to be apart from her parents—these are essential skills that your baby will take with her into adulthood.

I have seen couples—desperate, depressed, resentful, who feel as though they were sold some dream of parenthood that doesn't exist—turn into confident, satisfied, and well-rested parents. Their babies have transformed from being cranky, agitated, and "high needs" to being happy, secure, curious, and confident. This transformation changes the focus of childhood to one of healthy physical and psychological development rather than one of surviving sleep deprivation.

Rex: Out of the Car Seat and Into the Cot

Rex was 13 weeks old when his parents contacted me. I had worked with them 2 years before when they needed help teaching Rex's older brother to nap in the cot. Rex was napping fairly well, but he was always sleeping in a bouncy seat or car seat because he had reflux. He was outgrowing this, though, and clearly showing signs that he needed more space and mobility during the night.

Rex was going to bed too late, typically not until 8 or 9 p.m. He was feeding before getting his bath and then "topping off" during the bedtime routine. He was consistently falling asleep during that last minifeed but had to be held upright for a while because of the reflux. He was sleeping well for the first part of the night and then waking a couple of times to feed between midnight and 5 a.m. These feedings were becoming a problem because Rex was starting to become more physically uncomfortable with reflux. Rex's mother had the sense that he was overfeeding, making his reflux worse, but she was at a loss as to how to change it.

Rex's parents had been through cry-it-out with his brother, but they were worried that Rex was too young. Still, their family was showing strain because of the fatigue. Rex's mother was struggling with insomnia after his feedings, and she knew things couldn't go on like this.

Fortunately, Rex was not too young to cry it out. In fact, he really needed to stop feeding during the night because it was aggravating his reflux and disrupting his sleep. He was a big, otherwise healthy baby, and it was time to help him learn to self-soothe. We made some adjustments to the bedtime routine so that Rex could get to bed earlier. He stopped getting the extra minifeed during the bedtime routine. When his bedtime was moved earlier, Rex stopped falling asleep during the routine.

The first night of crying was the hardest. He cried in 30- to 40-minute bursts every hour or two. His parents had hoped he would get a longer stretch of sleep that first night, but the length of the crying episodes was much shorter than what they had experienced with their older son. The second night, Rex did not cry at bedtime, and he slept for several hours at a stretch, waking three times and crying—less intensely—for no more than 30 minutes each time. By the third night, he was down to one "annoying" waking around 4 a.m., but his parents couldn't remember how long he was awake (they were able to fall back to sleep). And after that, he slept like a champ.

My job is stressful and intense, but it is also incredibly gratifying. Parents put their trust in my knowledge and experience. And when I get notes in the mail or e-mails shouting "thank you" in all caps, I'm reminded of how fundamentally life changing it is for a family when a baby learns to sleep. Parents don't relish the memory of cry-it-out, but they don't regret having done it once they see how happy a well-rested baby—and family—can be.

Using extinction to teach infants to sleep is an emotional experience. Our instincts tell us that a crying baby needs our help. But a crying baby also needs to learn how to sleep. The best we can do is to try to separate our emotional experience from our job as parents. Science reassures us that we are doing the right thing even though it brings us all to tears.

The Good Sleeper Primer

Sleep is a popular topic, and most people I meet, whether socially or professionally, want to talk about what I do. Over the years, I have whittled down the way I describe my philosophy and approach to cover a few key points. You'll have to read the book to find the rationale and methods you'll need, but these rules of thumb sum up the main themes to take away.

1. You are the parent, and your baby needs you to be in charge.
2. Crying is not dangerous to your baby.
3. Overtired babies do not sleep well. Look for drowsiness cues and heed them.
4. Establish bedtime routines so your baby doesn't need to fall asleep while eating or being held.
5. Put your baby down in the cot.
6. Understand the basics of your baby's natural biorhythm and the role of melatonin in sleep. Work with your baby's sleep clock instead of against it.
7. Remember that infant sleep is different from adult sleep and that much of raising a good sleeper seems counterintuitive.
8. Keeping your baby awake to spend time with him is not good for him.
9. Teaching your baby to sleep is a lifelong *gift*.
10. Don't forget to take care of yourself, too.

Sleep Diaries

Infant Sleep Diary

DAY	SUNDAY	MONDAY
Date		
Time up		
Nap 1 routine		
Nap time/Duration		
Nap 2 routine		
Nap time/ Duration		
Nap 3 routine		
Nap time/Duration		
Bedtime routine (include start time)		
Time to sleep		
Waking #1 (time/intervention)		
Waking #2 (time/intervention)		
Other wakings		
Other notes		

TUESDAY	WEDNESDAY	THURSDAY	FRIDAY	SATURDAY

Adult Sleep Diary

Name:_____

DAY	(EXAMPLE)	
Naps	2–3 p.m.	
Exercise	5 p.m. × 30 min.	
Caffeine (coffee, tea, soda, chocolate)	10, 2 p.m. coffee	
Alcohol	1 wine, 7 p.m.	
Sleep Medication (time and dose)	5 mg Amb. 10 p.m.	
What time did you go to bed?	10:30 p.m.	
What time did you turn out the lights?	10:45 p.m.	
What time did you fall asleep?	11 p.m.	
How many times did you wake up during the night?	2	
Total length of interruptions (minutes)	15	
What time did you wake up (for the last time) in the morning?	6 a.m.	
What time did you get out of bed?	7:30 a.m.	
How many hours of sleep did you get (total)?	6.75	
How many hours did you spend in bed (total)?	9.00	
How sound was your sleep overall? (1 = very restless, 5 = very sound)	3	
How rested did you feel in the morning? (1 = exhausted, 5 = refreshed)	4	
Notes/Comments: (mood, activities, stress, etc.)		

Week _____ to _____

Index of Case Examples

Recommended Reading
and Viewing

The following sources have served as references in the writing of this book. They provide additional useful information and have informed my work.

Ferber, Richard. *Solve Your Child's Sleep Problems: New, Revised, and Expanded Edition.* New York: Simon and Schuster, 2006.
Dr. Ferber is essentially the father of sleep training as we know it. In addition to a detailed discussion of graduated-extinction methods, this book provides a comprehensive look at sleep development, sleep disorders, and parenting practices around sleep.

Karp, Harvey. *The Happiest Baby on the Block.* The Happiest Baby, Inc., 2012. DVD. 128 min.
This is essential viewing for every new parent. Dr. Karp demonstrates how to calm a fussy baby. This video will give you the tools you need to get through the fussy weeks with your sanity intact.

Mindell, Jodi A. *Sleeping Through the Night, Revised Edition: How Infants, Toddlers, and Their Parents Can Get a Good Night's Sleep.* New York: Morrow, 2005.

Dr. Mindell is a psychologist and sleep researcher whose work informs pediatric sleep-medicine standards of practice. *Sleeping Through the Night* provides excellent background on the behavioral and physical science of sleep medicine for the lay reader.

Moore, Polly. *The 90-Minute Baby Sleep Program: Follow Your Child's Natural Sleep Rhythms for Better Nights and Naps.* New York: Workman, 2008.

Dr. Moore, a neuroscientist, provides a detailed discussion of the neurological basis for the 90-minute window in this book. Although my methods and adherence to the 90-minute rule differ from her program, the scientific explanation of the process involved makes this a good resource for additional information.

Morin, Charles M., et al. *Insomnia.* New York: Wiley, 1993.

This book is written for clinicians treating insomnia in adults. It is the basis of my clinical work with adults and a reference point for the physical and behavioral science of insomnia.

Weissbluth, Marc. *Healthy Sleep Habits, Happy Child.* New York: Random House, 1999.

Healthy Sleep Habits, Happy Child is the book I read before my first child was born. It provides a thorough discussion of the science of sleep, infant sleep development, overfatigue and the value of keeping your baby well rested, and the rationale for using extinction methods.

References from Appendix A:
Cry-It-Out: Is It Harmful?

Ahnert, L., Gunnar, M. R., Lamb, M. E., and Barthel, M. "Transition to Child Care: Associations with Infant-Mother Attachment, Infant Negative Emotion, and Cortisol Elevations." *Child Development* 75, no. 3 (2004): 639–50.

Ainsworth, M. D. S., Blehar, M. C., Waters, E., and Wall, S. *Patterns of Attachment: A Psychological Study of the Strange Situation.* New York: Psychology Press, 2014.

Brazy, J. E. "Effects of Crying on Cerebral Blood Volume and Cytochrome *aa3.*" *The Journal of Pediatrics* 112, no. 3 (1988): 457–61.

Butler, S. R., Suskind, M. R., and Schanberg, S. M. "Maternal Behavior as a Regulator of Polyamine Biosynthesis in Brain and Heart of the Developing Rat Pup." *Science* 199, no. 4327 (1978): 445–47.

Coe, C. L., Wiener, S. G., Rosenberg, L. T., and Levine, S. "Endocrine and Immune Responses to Separation and Maternal Loss in Non-Human Primates." In *The Psychobiology of Attachment and Separation*, edited by M. Reite and T. Field, 163–99. Orlando: Academic Press, 1985.

Črnčec, R., Matthey, S., and Nemeth, D. "Infant Sleep Problems and Emotional Health: A Review of Two Behavioural Approaches." *Journal of Reproductive and Infant Psychology* 28, no. 1 (2010): 44–54.

de Weerth, C., and van Geert, P. "A Longitudinal Study of Basal Cortisol in Infants: Intra-individual Variability, Circadian Rhythm and Developmental Trends." *Infant Behavior and Development* 25, no. 4 (2002): 375–98.

France, K. G. "Behavior Characteristics and Security in Sleep-Disturbed Infants Treated with Extinction." *Journal of Pediatric Psychology* 17, no. 4 (1992): 467–75.

Gunnar, M. R., Brodersen, L., Krueger, K., and Rigatuso, J. "Dampening of Adrenocortical Responses During Infancy: Normative Changes and Individual Differences." *Child Development* 67, no. 3 (1996): 877–89.

Gunnar, M. R., Connors, J., Isensee, J., and Wall, L. "Adrenocortical Activity and Behavioral Distress in Human Newborns." *Developmental Psychobiology* 21, no. 4 (1988): 297–310.

Hiscock, H., and Wake, M. "Randomised Controlled Trial of Behavioural Infant Sleep Intervention to Improve Infant Sleep and Maternal Mood." *British Medical Journal* 324, no. 7345 (2002): 1062.

Hofer, M. A. "The Mother-Infant Interaction as a Regulator of Infant Physiology and Behavior." In *Symbiosis in Parent-Offspring Interactions*, edited by L. A. Rosenblum and H. Moltz, 61–75. New York: Springer US, 1983.

Hofer, M. A., and Shair, H. "Control of Sleep-Wake States in the Infant Rat by Features of the Mother-Infant Relationship." *Developmental Psychobiology* 15, no. 3 (1982): 229–43.

Hollenbeck, A. R., Susman, E. J., Nannis, E. D., Strope, B. E., Hersh, S. P., Levine, A. S., and Pizzo, P. A. "Children with Serious Illness: Behavioral Correlates of Separation and Isolation." *Child Psychiatry and Human Development* 11, no. 1 (1980): 3–11.

Kaufman, J., and Charney, D. "Effects of Early Stress on Brain Structure and Function: Implications for Understanding the Relationship Between Child Maltreatment and Depression." *Development and Psychopathology* 13, no. 3 (2001): 451–71.

Kuhn, C. M., and Schanberg, S. M. "Selective Depression of Serum Growth Hormone During Maternal Deprivation in Rat Pups." *Science* 201, no. 4360 (1978): 1034–36.

Larson, M. C., White, B. P., Cochran, A., Donzella, B., and Gunnar, M. "Dampening of the Cortisol Response to Handling at 3 Months in Human Infants and Its Relation to Sleep, Circadian Cortisol Activity, and Behavioral Distress." *Developmental Psychobiology* 33, no. 4 (1998): 327–37.

Lieberman, A. F., and Zeanah, C. H. "Disorders of Attachment in Infancy." *Child and Adolescent Psychiatric Clinics of North America* 4, no. 3 (1995): 571–87.

Ludington-Hoe, S. M., Cong, X., and Hashemi, F. "Infant Crying: Nature, Physiologic Consequences, and Select Interventions." *Neonatal Network: The Journal of Neonatal Nursing* 21, no. 2 (2002): 29–36.

Martins, C., and Gaffan, E. A. "Effects of Early Maternal Depression on Patterns of Infant-Mother Attachment: A Meta-Analytic Investigation." *Journal of Child Psychology and Psychiatry* 41, no. 6 (2000): 737–46.

Middlemiss, W., Granger, D. A., and Goldberg, W. A. "Response to 'Let's Help Parents Help Themselves: A Letter to the Editor Supporting the Safety of Behavioural Sleep Techniques.'" *Early Human Development* 89, no. 1 (2013): 41–42.

Middlemiss, W., Granger, D. A., Goldberg, W. A., and Nathans, L. "Asynchrony of Mother-Infant Hypothalamic-Pituitary-Adrenal Axis Activity Following Extinction of Infant Crying Responses Induced During the Transition to Sleep." *Early Human Development* 88, no. 4 (2012): 227–32.

Mindell, J. A., Kuhn, B., Lewin, D. S., Meltzer, L. J., and Sadeh, A. "Behavioral Treatment of Bedtime Problems and Night Wakings in Infants and Young Children." *Pediatric Sleep* 29, no. 10 (2006): 1263–76.

Narvaez, D. "Dangers of Crying It Out: Damaging Children and Their Relationships for the Longterm." http://www.psychologytoday.com/blog/moral-landscapes /201112/dangers-crying-it-out.

Perry, B. "Incubated in Terror: Neurodevelopmental Factors in the Cycle of Violence," In *Children in a Violent Society*, edited by J. D. Osofsky, 124–48. New York: Guilford Press, 1997.

Price, A. M. H., Wake, M., Ukoumunne, O. C., and Hiscock, H. "Five-year Follow-up of Harms and Benefits of Behavioral Infant Sleep Intervention: Randomized Trial." *Pediatrics* 130, no. 4 (2012): 643–51.

Rao, M. R., Brenner, R. A., Schisterman, E. F., Vik, T., and Mills, J. L. "Long Term Cognitive Development in Children with Prolonged Crying." *Archives of Disease in Childhood* 89, no. 11 (2004): 989–92.

Sears, W., Sears, M., Sears, R., and Sears, J. *The Baby Book: Everything You Need to Know About Your Baby from Birth to Age Two*. Rev. and updated ed. New York: Little, Brown, 2003.

———. *The Baby Book, Revised Edition: Everything You Need to Know About Your Baby from Birth to Age Two*. New York: Hachette Digital, Inc., 2013.

———. "Science Says: Excessive Crying Could Be Harmful." AskDrSears.com. http://www.askdrsears.com/topics/health-concerns/fussy-baby/science-says-excessive-crying-could-be-harmful.

Stifter, C. A., and Spinrad, T. L. "The Effect of Excessive Crying on the Development of Emotion Regulation." *Infancy* 3, no. 2 (2002): 133–52.

Teicher, M. H., Andersen, S. L., Polcari, A., Anderson, C. M., Navalta, C. P., and Kim, D. M. "The Neurobiological Consequences of Early Stress and Childhood

Maltreatment." *Neuroscience & Biobehavioral Reviews* 27, no. 1 (2003): 33–44.

Teti, D. M., Gelfand, D. M., Messinger, D. S., and Isabella, R. "Maternal Depression and the Quality of Early Attachment: An Examination of Infants, Pre-schoolers, and Their Mothers." *Developmental Psychology* 31, no. 3 (1995): 364.

Wolke, D., Rizzo, P., and Woods, S. "Persistent Infant Crying and Hyperactivity Problems in Middle Childhood." *Pediatrics* 109, no. 6 (2002): 1054–60.

Additional Sources

Ainsworth, M. D. S., Blehar, M. C., Waters, E., and Wall, S. *Patterns of Attachment: A Psychological Study of the Strange Situation*. New York: Psychology Press, 2014.

Attanasio, A., Borrelli, P., and Gupta, D. "Circadian Rhythms in Serum Melatonin from Infancy to Adolescence." *The Journal of Clinical Endocrinology & Metabolism* 61, no. 2 (1985): 388–90.

Babyak, M., Blumenthal, J. A., Herman, S., Khatri, P., Doraiswamy, M., Moore, K., . . . and Krishnan, K. R. "Exercise Treatment for Major Depression: Maintenance of Therapeutic Benefit at 10 Months." *Psychosomatic Medicine* 62, no. 5 (2000): 633–38.

Ball, T. M., Castro-Rodriguez, J. A., Griffith, K. A., Holberg, C. J., Martinez, F. D., and Wright, A. L. "Siblings, Day-care Attendance, and the Risk of Asthma and Wheezing During Childhood." *New England Journal of Medicine* 343, no. 8 (2000): 538–43.

Ball, T. M., Holberg, C. J., Aldous, M. B., Martinez, F. D., and Wright, A. L. "Influence of Attendance at Day Care on the Common Cold from Birth Through 13 Years of Age." *Archives of Pediatrics & Adolescent Medicine* 156, no. 2 (2002): 121–26.

Barr, R. G. "Changing Our Understanding of Infant Colic." *Archives of Pediatrics & Adolescent Medicine* 156, no. 12 (2002): 1172–74.

Blair, P. S., Fleming, P. J., Smith, I. J., Platt, M. W., Young, J., Nadin, P., . . . and Mitchell, E. "Babies Sleeping with Parents: Case-control Study of Factors Influencing the Risk of the Sudden Infant Death Syndrome. Commentary: Cot Death—the Story So Far." *British Medical Journal* 319, no. 7223 (1999): 1457–62.

Blumenthal, J. A., Babyak, M. A., Doraiswamy, P. M., Watkins, L., Hoffman, B. M., Barbour, K. A., . . . and Sherwood, A. "Exercise and Pharmacotherapy in the Treatment of Major Depressive Disorder." *Psychosomatic Medicine* 69, no. 7 (2007): 587–96.

Carpenter, R. G., Irgens, L. M., Blair, P. S., England, P. D., Fleming, P., Huber, J., . . . and Schreuder, P. "Sudden Unexplained Infant Death in 20 Regions in Europe: Case Control Study." *The Lancet* 363, no. 9404 (2004): 185–91.

Claustrat, B., Brun, J., and Chazot, G. "The Basic Physiology and Pathophysiology of Melatonin." *Sleep Medicine Reviews* 9, no. 1 (2005): 11–24.

Clifford, T. J., Campbell, M. K., Speechley, K. N., and Gorodzinsky, F. "Sequelae of Infant Colic: Evidence of Transient Infant Distress and Absence of Lasting Effects on Maternal Mental Health." *Archives of Pediatrics & Adolescent Medicine* 156, no. 12 (2002): 1183–88.

Colrain, I. M., and Campbell, K. B. "The Use of Evoked Potentials in Sleep Research." *Sleep Medicine Reviews* 11, no. 4 (2007): 277–93.

Cote, K. A. "Probing Awareness During Sleep with the Auditory Odd-Ball Paradigm." *International Journal of Psychophysiology* 46, no. 3 (2002): 227–41.

Demo, D. H., and Cox, M. J. "Families with Young Children: A Review of Research in the 1990s." *Journal of Marriage and Family* 62, no. 4 (2000): 876–95.

de Weerth, C., Zijl, R. H., and Buitelaar, J. K. "Development of Cortisol Circadian Rhythm in Infancy." *Early Human Development* 73, no. 1 (2003): 39–52.

Dunn, A. L., Trivedi, M. H., Kampert, J. B., Clark, C. G., and Chambliss, H. O. "Exercise Treatment for Depression: Efficacy and Dose Response." *American Journal of Preventive Medicine* 28, no. 1 (2005): 1–8.

Garrison, M. M., and Christakis, D. A. "A Systematic Review of Treatments for Infant Colic." *Pediatrics* 106, supplement 1 (2000): 184–90.

Gaylor, E. E., Burnham, M. M., Goodlin-Jones, B. L., and Anders, T. F. "A Longitudinal Follow-up Study of Young Children's Sleep Patterns Using a Developmental Classification System." *Behavioral Sleep Medicine* 3, no. 1 (2005): 44–61.

Hauck, F. R., Herman, S. M., Donovan, M., Iyasu, S., Moore, C. M., Donoghue, E., . . . and Willinger, M. "Sleep Environment and the Risk of Sudden Infant Death Syndrome in an Urban Population: The Chicago Infant Mortality Study." *Pediatrics* 111, supplement 1 (2003): 1207–14.

Iglowstein, I., Jenni, O. G., Molinari, L., and Largo, R. H. "Sleep Duration from Infancy to Adolescence: Reference Values and Generational Trends." *Pediatrics* 111, no. 2 (2003): 302–7.

Jacobsen, T., and Hofmann, V. "Children's Attachment Representations: Longitudinal Relations to School Behavior and Academic Competency in Middle Childhood and Adolescence." *Developmental Psychology* 33, no. 4 (1997): 703.

Kennaway, D. J., Stamp, G. E., and Goble, F. C. "Development of Melatonin Production in Infants and the Impact of Prematurity." *The Journal of Clinical Endocrinology and Metabolism* 75, no. 2 (1992): 367–69.

Meerlo, P., Sgoifo, A., and Suchecki, D. "Restricted and Disrupted Sleep: Effects on Autonomic Function, Neuroendocrine Stress Systems and Stress Responsivity." *Sleep Medicine Reviews* 12, no. 3 (2008): 197–210.

Miller, A. R., and Barr, R. G. "Infantile Colic. Is It a Gut Issue?" *Pediatric Clinics of North America* 38, no. 6 (1991): 1407–23.

Mindell, J. A., Meltzer, L. J., Carskadon, M. A., and Chervin, R. D. "Developmental Aspects of Sleep Hygiene: Findings from the 2004 National Sleep Foundation 'Sleep in America Poll.' " *Sleep Medicine* 10, no. 7 (2009): 771–79.

Moore, D. J., Tao, B. S. K., Lines, D. R., Hirte, C., Heddle, M. L., and Davidson, G. P. "Double-Blind Placebo-Controlled Trial of Omeprazole in Irritable Infants with Gastroesophageal Reflux." *The Journal of Pediatrics* 143, no. 2 (2003): 219–23.

Morin, C. M., and Espie, C. A., eds. *Insomnia: A Clinician's Guide to Assessment and Treatment*, vol. 1. New York: Springer, 2003.

Mullington, J. M., Haack, M., Toth, M., Serrador, J. M., and Meier-Ewert, H. K. "Cardiovascular, Inflammatory, and Metabolic Consequences of Sleep Deprivation." *Progress in Cardiovascular Diseases* 51, no. 4 (2009): 294–302.

National Sleep Foundation: http://sleepfoundation.org/sleep-topics/children-and-sleep.

Neal, J., and Frick-Horbury, D. "The Effects of Parenting Styles and Childhood Attachment Patterns on Intimate Relationships." *Journal of Instructional Psychology* 28, no. 3 (2001): 178–83.

Nicolaou, N. C., Simpson, A., Lowe, L. A., Murray, C. S., Woodcock, A., and Custovic, A. "Day-Care Attendance, Position in Sibship, and Early Childhood Wheezing: A Population-Based Birth Cohort Study." *Journal of Allergy and Clinical Immunology* 122, no. 3 (2008): 500–506.

Pavlov, I. P. *Conditioned Reflexes*. London: Oxford University Press, 1927.

Pharoah, P. "Bed-Sharing and Sudden Infant Death." *The Lancet* 347, no. 8993 (1996): 2.

Pinilla, T., and Birch, L. L. "Help Me Make It Through the Night: Behavioral Entrainment Breast-Fed Infants' Sleep Patterns." *Pediatrics* 91, no. 2 (1993): 436–44.

Price, D. A., Close, G. C., and Fielding, B. A. "Age of Appearance of Circadian Rhythm in Salivary Cortisol Values in Infancy." *Archives of Disease in Childhood* 58, no. 6 (1983): 454–56.

Rivkees, S. A. "Developing Circadian Rhythmicity in Infants." *Pediatrics* 112, no. 2 (2003): 373–81.

Santiago, L. B., Jorge, S. M., and Moreira, A. C. "Longitudinal Evaluation of the Development of Salivary Cortisol Circadian Rhythm in Infancy." *Clinical Endocrinology* 44, no. 2 (1996): 157–61.

Scherer, L. D., Zikmund-Fisher, B. J., Fagerlin, A., and Tarini, B. A. "Influence of 'GERD' Label on Parents' Decision to Medicate Infants." *Pediatrics* 131, no. 5 (2013): 839–45.

Scragg, R. K. R., Stewart, A. W., Mitchell, E. A., Thompson, J. M. D., Taylor, B. J., Williams, S. M., and Hassall, I. B. "Infant Room-Sharing and Prone Sleep Position in Sudden Infant Death Syndrome." *The Lancet* 347, no. 8993 (1996): 7–12.

Skinner, B. F. "A Case History in Scientific Method." *American Psychologist* 11 (1956): 221–33.

Stevens, R. G., Brainard, G. C., Blask, D. E., Lockley, S. W., and Motta, M. E. "Adverse Health Effects of Nighttime Lighting: Comments on American Medical Association Policy Statement." *American Journal of Preventive Medicine* 45, no. 3 (2013): 343–46.

Tappin, D., Ecob, R., and Brooke, H. "Bedsharing, Roomsharing, and Sudden Infant Death Syndrome in Scotland: A Case-Control Study." *The Journal of Pediatrics* 147, no. 1 (2005): 32–37.

Task Force on Sudden Infant Death Syndrome. "SIDS and Other Sleep-Related Infant Deaths: Expansion of Recommendations for a Safe Infant Sleeping Environment." *Pediatrics* 128 (2011): 1341–67.

Tinanoff, N., and O'Sullivan, D. M. "Early Childhood Caries: Overview and Recent Findings." *Pediatric Dentistry* 19 (1997): 12–16.

Touchette, É., Petit, D., Paquet, J., Boivin, M., Japel, C., Tremblay, R. E., and Montplaisir, J. Y. "Factors Associated with Fragmented Sleep at Night across Early Childhood." *Archives of Pediatrics and Adolescent Medicine* 159, no. 3 (2005): 242–49.

Waldhauser, F., and Reiter, E. "Age-Related Changes in Melatonin Levels in Humans and Its Potential Consequences for Sleep Disorders." *Experimental Gerontology* 33, no. 7 (1998): 759–72.

Waldhauser, F., Weiszenbacher, G., Tatzer, E., Gisinger, B., Waldhauser, M., Schemper, M., and Frisch, H. "Alterations in Nocturnal Serum Melatonin Levels in Humans with Growth and Aging." *The Journal of Clinical Endocrinology & Metabolism* 66, no. 3 (1988): 648–52.

Wessel, M. A., Cobb, J. C., Jackson, E. B., Harris, G. S., and Detwiler, A. C. "Paroxysmal Fussing in Infancy, Sometimes Called 'Colic.'" *Pediatrics* 14, no. 5 (1954): 421–35.

Acknowledgments

I am incredibly grateful to my excellent editor, Serena Jones, for seeking me out after attending my Raise a Good Sleeper class and for convincing me that the time was right for this book done in this way. It also helped that she introduced me to my agent and worked some kind of magic to bring the book to Holt.

To my agent, Meg Thompson, and everyone at Einstein Thompson Agency, my sincerest thanks. Meg's support and hard bargaining allowed me the time and space to devote to doing this right.

Thanks to Dr. Michel Cohen for turning a chance encounter on the street into a years-long gig teaching my Raise a Good Sleeper class at his medical offices. And to

Erica Lyon, director of Pregnancy and Parenting, for her continued support for the class and this book.

I want to thank Britt Ahlstrom for her thorough literature searching and cataloguing of essential citations that gave me a huge jump start on researching the real data on sleep training. I also thank James Kemp, MD, for being my point person on infant sleep safety and for his enthusiasm about this project.

I thank Karen Massie, my high school English teacher, for training me to write confidently, concisely, and efficiently.

I have received tremendous support from my family and friends, among them my brother and brother-in-law, Larry Krone and Jim Andralis; my parents, Ann and Ron Krone; Dave, Amy, Linda, Leonida; and Eleanor Safe, forever my soul sister.

Thank you to Maryhope Howland Rutherford and Christie Pfaff, both psychologists and mums, for their insightful comments, which made this a better book.

To Erin St. John Kelly, a very talented writer-editor whose hours of investment, line edits, and keen eye for emphasis gave me needed energy at the end of an exhausting run, I thank you, my dear friend.

To my amazing son and daughter who have inspired me to make them proud.

To my husband, Randy, who has believed in me from the start and has encouraged me at every stage of my education and career, thank you for buying my URL to cheer me up after an especially bad day at the hospital, for nodding slowly in baffled agreement when I declared that we would be taking out a home equity loan to start my business at the beginning of the recession, for always making my personal and professional fulfillment a priority in our partnership, and for being a wonderful dad.

And to the hundreds of parents who have invited me into their families, often during very dark times, and trusted me to help them raise good sleepers. It is an honor to do this incredibly fulfilling work and to be a part of so many wonderful people's lives.

Index